Cell Adhesion and Cytoskeletal Molecules in Metastasis

Cancer Metastasis – Biology and Treatment

VOLUME 9

Recent Volumes in this Series

Volume 4: Proteases and Their Inhibitors in Cancer Metastasis
Editor: Jean-Michel Foidart and Ruth J. Muschel
ISBN 1-4020-0923-2

Volume 5: Micrometastasis
Editor: Klaus Pantel
ISBN 1-4020-1155-5

Volume 6: Bone Metastasis and Molecular Mechanisms
Editors: Gurmit Singh and William Orr
ISBN 1-4020-1984-X

Volume 7: DNA Methylation, Epigenetics and Metastasis
Editor: Manel Esteller
ISBN 1-4020-3641-8

Volume 8: Cell Motility in Cancer Invasion and Metastasis
Editor: Alan Wells
ISBN 1-4020-4008-3

Cell Adhesion and Cytoskeletal Molecules in Metastasis

Edited by

Anne E. Cress
University of Arizona, Tucson, AZ, U.S.A.

and

Raymond B. Nagle
University of Arizona, Tucson, AZ, U.S.A.

Springer

A C.I.P. Catalogue record for this book is available from the Library of Congress.

ISBN-10 1-4020-5128-X (HB)
ISBN-13 978-1-4020-5128-9 (HB)
ISBN-10 1-4020-5129-8 (e-book)
ISBN-13 978-1-4020-5129-6 (e-book)

Published by Springer,
P.O. Box 17, 3300 AA Dordrecht, The Netherlands.

www.springer.com

Printed on acid-free paper

TABLE OF CONTENTS

LIST OF CONTRIBUTORS

Nelson R. Alexander
Department of Surgery and the Cancer Biology GraduateProgram, Arizona Health Sciences Center, University of Arizona, Tucson, AZ, USA

Elisabeth L. Bair
Department of Pathology, Arizona Cancer Center, University of Arizona, Tucson, AZ, USA

Sanjay Chauhan
Department of Biochemistry and Molecular Biophysics, University of Arizona, Tucson, AZ, USA

Ryan Childers
Department of Biochemistry and Molecular Biophysics, University of Arizona, Tucson, AZ, USA

Nils Cordes
OcoRay-Radiation Research in Oncology, Medical Faculty Carl Gustav Carus, University of Technology, Dresden, Germany

Anne E. Cress
Department of Cell Biology and Anatomy, Arizona Cancer Center, University of Arizona, Tucson, AZ, USA

Tracy L. Davis
Department of Pathology, Massachusetts General Hospital, Boston, Massachusetts, USA

Frederick E. Domann
Free Radical and Radiation Biology Program, Department of Radiation Oncology, Carver College of Medicine and Holden Cancer Center, University of Iowa, Iowa City, IA, USA

Aaron J. Goldman
Department of Molecular and Cellular Biology, University of Arizona, Tucson, Arizona, USA

Bernard W. Futscher
Department of Pharmacology and Toxicology, College of Pharmacy, Arizona Cancer Center, University of Arizona, Tucson, AZ, USA

Lori A. Hazlehurst
H. Lee Moffitt Cancer Center & Research Institute, University of South Florida, Tampa, FL, USA

Ronald L. Heimark
Department of Surgery and the Cancer Biology GraduateProgram, Arizona Health Sciences Center, University of Arizona, Tucson, AZ, USA

Jennifer Himes
Departments of Biochemistry and Molecular Biophysics, University of Arizona, Tucson, AZ, USA

Susan Kunz
Departments of Biochemistry and Molecular Biophysics, University of Arizona, Tucson, AZ, USA

Kit S. Lam
University of California Davis Cancer Center, Division of Hematology/Oncology and the Department of Internal Medicine, University of California, Davis, CA, USA

Roger L. Miesfeld
Department of Biochemistry and Molecular Biophysics, Department of Molecular and Cellular Biology, University of Arizona, Tucson, AZ, USA

Raymond B. Nagle
Arizona Cancer Center, University of Arizona, Tucson, AZ, USA

Anil Prasad
Department of Pathology, Southern Arizona Veterans Affairs Health Care System, and Department of Pathology, Arizona Health Sciences Center, University of Arizona, Tucson, AZ, USA

Andrea Pierce
Departments of Biochemistry and Molecular Biophysics, University of Arizona, Tucson, AZ, USA

Kelvin W. Pond
Arizona Cancer Center, University of Arizona, Tucson, AZ, USA

Isaac Rabinovitz
Department of Pathology, Beth Israel Deaconess Medical Center and Harvard Medical School, Boston, MA, USA

Monika Schmelz
Department of Pathology, Southern Arizona Veterans Affairs Health Care System, and Department of Pathology, Arizona Health Sciences Center, University of Arizona, Tucson, AZ, USA

Kaylene J. Simpson
Department of Cell Biology, Harvard Medical School, Boston, MA, USA

Sabrina Sykes
Department of Biochemistry and Molecular Biophysics, University of Arizona, Tucson, AZ, USA

Thomas C. Sroka
Arizona Cancer Center, University of Arizona, Tucson, AZ, USA

FOREWORD

The ability of an epithelial cell to adhere to its neighbor and to the extracellular environment is an essential process that defines in part, a normal multicellular organism. It is a feature that is fundamental to the development of an organism. Mutations in critical adhesion components will result either in embryonic lethal phenotypes at various stages or lethality shortly after birth. In addition, adhesion structures are essential for the survival of the adult organism, as mutations will also result in defective wound healing responses in a variety of organ systems.

Although many adhesion structures exist that are required for successful epithelial cell adhesion, the focus of this volume is to highlight the necessity for the transformed epithelial cell to adhere either to the extracellular environment via integrin type receptors or to adhere to its neighbor through cadherin complexes during tumor progression. The alteration of the requirements of cellular adhesion during tumor progression and metastasis is the subject of Chapters 1-3.

Cell adhesion structures are normally tightly regulated but their components are corrupted for nepharious purposes such as cancer cell invasion, migration and attachment at a distant site. The cytoskeleton is involved in these processes. In Chapter 4, the actin cytoskeleton and integrin receptors normally engaged in strong stable adhesion structures are discussed as migration determinants. In Chapter 5, a FERM domain protein, known to interact with F-actin, called EHM2, is discussed as a metastasis promoting agent. In Chapter 6, the cytokeratin 6 network of the cytoskeleton is postulated as a critical element in the maturation of a stem cell component within a normal prostate gland.

The molecules involved in cell adhesion structures are uniquely positioned to serve as membrane sentinels for the changing extracellular environment of a metastatic cell. This is an important requirement of a metastatic cancer cell to survive the dynamic environments encountered during intravasation and extravasation, prior to reaching a distant site. In Chapter 7, the epigenetic regulation of cell adhesion genes is discussed as a potential mechanism to confer transient suppression of cell adhesion genes during the metastatic process. The ability of cell adhesion structures to influence damage responses through the action of cell surface receptors is detailed in Chapters 8 and 9.

The reliance of the cancer cell upon cell adhesion for invasion, migration and survival during and after the journey to a distant site makes it formally possible to block these events using small peptide extracellular adhesion mimetics. Chapter 10 illustrates the potential for generating and targeting epithelial cell surfaces using synthetic D-amino acid peptides.

The reliance of the metastatic cancer cell on a restricted set of adhesion structures derived from normal structures offers the opportunity for the early identification and eradication of circulating tumor cells with a pro-survival and pro-metastatic phenotype. Understanding the minimum elements of the adhesion structures that are selected for and preserved on the cancer cell during tumor progression will offer the possibility of defining adhesion receptors that dictate the metastatic adhesion signature. Stated another way, the metastatic adhesion signature confers an advantage for cancer cell survival and adhesion at the metastatic site; this reveals a potential vulnerability of the successful metastatic cell. Future work defining the metastatic adhesion structure(s) is likely to lead to improved early detection and prevention of cancer metastasis.

Anne E. Cress
Raymond B. Nagle
Arizona Cancer Center,
University of Arizona,
Tucson, AZ, USA

Chapter 1

CHANGING EXTRACELLULAR MATRIX LIGANDS DURING METASTASIS

Elisabeth L. Bair and Raymond B. Nagle
Arizona Cancer Center, University of Arizona, Tucson, AZ, USA

Abstract: Cellular homeostasis is achieved by cells continuously sending and receiving information, through cell-cell contacts, signals from the surrounding extracellular matrix (ECM), or from soluble hormones and growth factors. During cancer progression, these normal signals may be altered in a variety of ways forcing extracellular and intracellular changes to occur that will favor metastasis. Altering ECM ligands is a major mechanism by which transformed cells metastasize. One way in which ECM ligands change is through alterations in ECM composition. Another mechanism is through proteolysis of ECM proteins causing the release of growth factors or cryptic ECM peptides called matrikines. In this chapter, we will discuss changes that occur in ECM and examine how these changes are important for successful cancer metastasis.

Key words: extracellular matrix; matrikine; protease; cell adhesion molecules

1. ORGANIZATION OF THE EXTRACELLULAR MATRIX

The extracellular matrix (ECM) is a complex network of proteins surrounding cells, serving as a structural element in tissues. The ECM provides cells with information about their environment and thus influences tissue development. The basal lamina (BL) which surrounds epithelial cells is a highly structured, specialized form of ECM. The BL is a component of the basement membrane (BM), and are thin, specialized forms of ECM that surround muscle, fat, peripheral nerve cells, and all epithelial and endothelial cells (1). The ECM also includes the interstitium, which surrounds connective tissue cells and separate islets of epithelial cells.

A.E. Cress and R.B. Nagle (eds.), Cell Adhesion and Cytoskeletal Molecules in Metastasis, 1–18.

BLs are responsible for tissue compartmentalization, acting as a barrier for cells. BLs are found at the dermal-epidermal junction of skin; at the base of all lumen-lining epithelia of the digestive, respiratory, reproductive, and urinary tracts; underlying capillary endothelium and venules; around Schwann cells in the nervous system; surrounding fat cells, skeletal muscle, and cardiac muscle cells; and at the base of parenchymal cells of exocrine and endocrine glands.

The BL varies to some extent from tissue to tissue based on which matrix proteins are secreted by surrounding cells, but its basic components include: collagen, elastin, proteoglycans, and "anchorage" proteins such as laminin, fibronectin, vitronectin, and entactin that serve as attachment sites for epithelial cells (2, 3). Other ECM components that modulate cell-matrix interactions include thrombospondin, tenascin, and osteonectin. The BL consists of two networks that can self-assemble independently of each other and are then connected by entactin (3-5). The first network is formed by laminins, which assemble through N-terminal interactions of the three short arms and give dynamic flexibility to the BL and signals that lead to cell polarization. The second network consists of type IV collagens and gives structural stability to the BL. The BL components are well-conserved throughout evolution, indicating the importance of correct BL proteins for the development of multicellular life.

1.1 Laminin

Laminins (LM) are a family of large (400-600 kDa) cross-shaped heterotrimers composed of an α, β, and γ chain that are each separate gene products. LMs are secreted by epithelial cells, endothelial cells, myoblasts, and monocytes. Self-assembly of LM isoforms into a network occurs when the three short arms interact via the N-terminal globular domains (LN modules) (6).

Currently, there are sixteen different LMs described in tissues (7), with five α, three β, and three γ chains identified, and a theoretical possibility for up to forty-five different trimers; indicating that it is likely that new chain combinations have yet to be discovered. However, certain chains are never seen paired with each other, so the actual number of combinations is probably much smaller (8, 9). LM is involved in cell adhesion, migration, differentiation, and neurite outgrowth. Each LM trimer is thought to transmit a unique set of signals to a cell, as a genetic knock-out of each LM chain in mice exhibit unique phenotypes (8).

1.2 Fibronectin

In the ECM, fibronectin exists as an insoluble glycoprotein. It is a 450kDa disulfide-linked rod-like dimer composed of three types of homologous, repeating modules (Types I – III). Fibronectin is synthesized by fibroblasts, myoblasts, and endothelial cells. Fibronectin is important for cell adhesion and interactions with collagens, heparin sulfate, and hyaluronic acid. It is also involved in cell spreading, movement, and proliferation. Fibronection can have effects on cellular differentiation as well (10).

1.3 Collagen

Collagen is the most abundant protein in the body. At least fourteen types of collagen have been identified, each type occurring in different locations throughout the body. Collagens are mainly secreted by fibroblasts, although some epithelial cells secrete collagens as well. Assembly mainly occurs outside of the cell after procollagen is formed intracellularly and secreted. Procollagen fibrils come together to form tropocollagen, and finally collagen is formed (11).

1.4 Proteoglycans

Proteoglycans are large (typically 250 kDa and 300nm in length) complex macromolecules composed of a core protein and multiple glycosaminoglycans (GAG) chains. Most proteoglycans are secreted as complete molecules by all cell types. The GAGs are repeating dissacharide units of sugar residues extended into long chains. Proteoglycans occupy a large hydrodynamic volume and they provide a "cushioning" mechanism to the extracellular space. Heparin sulfate containing proteoglycans are found anchored to the plasma membrane of almost all cell types. This anchorage occurs through interactions with proteoglycan receptors and is important for cell adhesion (12).

2. NORMAL FUNCTION OF THE EXTRACELLULAR MATRIX

Almost all mammalian cells are in contact with an ECM. Initially, the ECM was thought of as a simple "glue" that held cells together by providing structural support for tissues. Today, however, it is known that the ECM is more dynamic than "glue" and plays key roles in development through interactions with cell adhesion molecules (CAMs) on the cell surface (1). The type of matrix secreted and its components also change in various disease states. Mutated BL proteins can lead to diseases such as muscular dystrophies, epidermolysis bullosa, or cancer (13-15) further indicating the functional importance of BL as more than providing structure.

While the structural support the ECM provides is important, the proteins that make up the ECM vary from tissue to tissue, and this difference appears to provide signals for tissue differentiation (16). The ECM elicits effects on cell function through activation of signaling molecules such as Rho, ILK, FAK, Shc, Jnk (17-19). Different ECM molecules interact with different cell adhesion molecules to mediate a wide variety of cellular processes including growth, survival, differentiation, and migration (20, 21). Even exogenously reconstituted BMs can stimulate specific differentiation of a variety of cell types, including mammary cells, hepatocytes, endothelial cells, Sertoli cells, and Schwann cells (22-27).

ECM protein composition and CAM-ECM interaction changes can lead to apoptosis, which is important for processes such as development to occur (28). ECM proteins must turnover and degrade in order to illicit new signal transduction cascades during embryogenesis and in wound healing in the adult (29). This turnover is achieved through the function of proteolytic enzymes, such as matrix metalloproteinases (MMPs), which will be described later. ECM structures serve another important function as well; they act as a "sieving" mechanism for transport of nutrients, cellular metabolic products, and migratory cells (e.g., lymphocytes).

3. THE ECM IN CANCER

Cues from the extracellular environment are of key importance in determining a cell's fate. It is only logical that a similar process occurs during cancer progression, and that as a normal cell becomes cancerous, the extracellular environment provides it with cues for survival. The behavior of neoplastic cells cannot be understood without taking into account their active and reciprocal dialogue with their surroundings. Neoplastic cells interact with their extracellular environment similarly to normal cells. The difference is that cancer cells do not respond to the extracellular environment in the same way as a normal cell.

The ECM forms the substrate on which cancer cells proliferate and provides a partial barrier to their migration. During cancer progression the ECM is extensively modified and remodeled by proteases either secreted by neoplastic and non-neoplastic cells or localized at the surface of cells. As a result of the activity of these proteases, important changes in cell-cell and cell-ECM interactions occur, and new signals are generated from the cell surface (30, 31). This signaling affects gene expression and ultimately influences critical cell behaviors such as proliferation, survival, and motility. As cancer migrates from its original site, CAM protein expression by the cancer cell changes, allowing for different signaling pathways to be activated. ECM protein expression also changes, further altering cellular signaling, and proteolytic enzymes overexpressed by cancer cells or surrounding stromal cells break down extracellular matrix proteins. Changes in ECM protein, CAM and proteolytic enzyme expression during prostate cancer progression are outlined in Table 1 (32). This degradation can mediate migration in at least three different ways: degrading the ECM for a migration path, releasing sequestered growth factors, and release of ECM growth promoting cryptic protein domains, called matrikines. All of these processes promote cancer cell survival and are variations on normal processes (such as wound healing and growth) that occur in normal tissue.

Table 1. Changes in ECM related protein expression during human prostate cancer progression

	Normal	**Prostatic Intraepithelial Neoplasia**	**Cancer**
ECM Proteins	Ln-111,-121	Ln-111,-121	
	Ln-211	Ln-211	Ln-211
	Ln-332	Ln-332	
	Ln-511	Ln-511	Ln-511
	Collagen IV, α1,2,3,5,6	Collagen IV α1,2,3,5,6	Collagen IV α1,2,3
	Collagen VII	Collagen VII	
	Entactin	Entactin	Entactin
			Hyaluronic Acid
CAMS	Integrin α1,2,3,4,5,6,v β1	Integrin α1,2,3,4,6,v β1	Integrin α3,6 β1
	Integrin α6β4		
	E-cadherin	E-cadherin	EN-cadherin
Proteases		MT1-MMP	MT1-MMP
		MMP-7	MMP-7

Most, if not all cancers, acquire the same set of ectopic functions during their development: enhancement of growth signaling during hyperplasia and dysplasia, tissue invasion, enriched angiogenesis, and metastasis. Each of these steps represents an evasion of normal regulation in cells and tissues. A coordinated response among ECM proteins, proteolytic enzymes, CAMs, growth factors and cytokines must exist for a cancer cell to metastasize successfully. CAMs respond to the extracellular environment initiating responses in cancer cells that lead first to modulation of the extracellular environment by proteolysis of ECM proteins and second to induction of invasion through the BM. CAMs interact with the changed components of the BL causing a variety of signaling pathways to be activated. Some of these signals result in increased production of proteolytic enzymes to further change the BM and by signaling for changes in the expression of CAMs to allow the cell to become more motile. Understanding these events may lead to improved diagnostics and prognostics, and eventually to better treatment for advanced cancers.

4. EXPRESSION DURING CANCER PROGRESSION

During cellular differentiation, ECM proteins direct cells to differentiate into specialized cells. Various ECM proteins affect cells differently. Changes in matrix protein expression occur to alter ECM protein composition. ECM composition is altered in cancer progression, although it is not entirely clear how these alterations in ECM protein expression occur. Desmoplasia of tumors is a prime example of cancer cells modifying their extracellular environment. Desmoplasia occurs in many carcinomas, but is particularly prevelant in breast cancers. It is a stromal response to growth factors such as transforming growth factor-α (TGF-α), TGF-β, insulin-like growth factor (IGF-1), IGF-II, and platelet-derived growth factor (PDGF) secreted by cancer cells, in which fibroblasts in the interstitium are stimulated to secrete collagen (33-37). The secreted collagen forms a dense mass surrounding invasive breast cancers. Currently, it is not clear whether this desmoplastic response promotes or impedes breast cancer progression. Another way in which cancer cells modify their environment is through secreting their own ECM proteins, overriding the normal cell's ECM to form a new, more migratory matrix.

In addition to stromal-induced ECM modifications, neoplastic cells do have receptors for and/or can produce certain components of the matrix. This is well described for LMs, and the LMs become incorporated into matrix surrounding cancer cells (38). In addition to LM expression, evidence indicates that proteoglycan expression by cancer cells also promotes tumor progression (12). This capability to express matrix proteins enables them to bind to vascular endothelium and may be involved in their ability to metastasize. Cancer cells that secrete ECM proteins tend to secrete LM proteins, and certain LM such as laminin-α3β3γ2 (LM-332) and laminin-α5β1γ1 (LM-511), formerly called LM-5 and LM-10, respectively (7), tend to promote a more migratory phenotype than other LMs (39, 40). LM-332 has been shown to be expressed at the leading edge of invasive epithelial carcinomas, at the tumor-stromal interface of their leading edge (41). It is thought that cancer cells may secrete LM-332 for the sole purpose of laying down a path of laminin proteins for migration. Another way cancer cells modify their extracellular environment is through downregulation of certain ECM proteins. In cancer, fibronectin or fibronectin receptor (α5β1 integrin) levels tend to be reduced and this reduction is correlated with increased tumor growth. Conversely, reintroduction of fibronectin or α5β1 integrin into cells reverses this phenotype (42). In fact, LM-332 expression is lost in prostate cancer and reduced in breast cancer (43, 44). In breast, the γ2 chain of LM-332 is expressed and secreted in a monomeric form (44) and presumably this may be true for other epithelial cancers as well. Thus, the matrix surrounding cancer cells oftentimes differs from the ECM composition surrounding normal cells. The difference in ECM proteins expressed in normal human prostate and prostate cancer is demonstrated in Figure 1. This altered ECM will form new cell-matrix adhesion with cancer cells, thereby activating different signaling pathways, and coordinating different cellular processes.

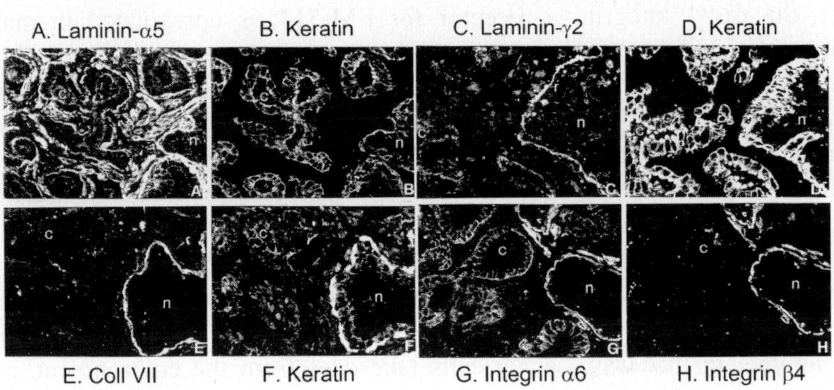

Figure 1. ECM protein expression in normal prostate and prostate cancer. Immunohistochemical analysis of human prostate tissue incubated with antibodies against ECM proteins and CAMs. A) Laminin-511 expression in both normal (n) and cancer (c), B) Keratin expression in n and c, C) Laminin-332 expression in n with downregulation in c, D) keratin expression in the same section as panel C, E) Collagen VII expression in n, with downregulation in c, F) keratin expression in same section as panel E, G) integrin α6 expression in n and c, and G) integrin β4 expression in the same section as panel G, demonstrating expression in n and disregulation in c. (Reprinted from Am J Pathol, 164:1211-1223, 2004 with permission from the American Society for Investigative Pathology).

5. ALTERED ADHESION MOLECULE EXPRESSION DURING CANCER PROGRESSION

CAMs such as integrins and cadherins are the proteins responsible for initializing extracellular signals. CAMs interact with the extracellular environment, and by attaching to other cells or ECM proteins, they transmit cues from the outer environment so that cells can activate necessary cellular processes for survival (16, 45). Depending on which type of ECM proteins are present, certain CAMs will bind to the ECM. Studies of integrins in transformed cells suggest that various integrin subunits may contribute either positively or negatively to the transformed cell phenotype (46). If a ligand for CAMs expressed by normal cells is not present in the ECM surrounding cancer, there is no reason for that cell to produce it. Therefore, it may turn off expression of unnecessary CAMs.

In addition, cancer cells may upregulate the expression of CAMs that will interact with their extracellular environment. This, in turn, can promote cues for metastasis. For example, a cancer cell secreting LM-511 will express CAMs that interact with LM-511, and those CAMs transmit promigratory signals into the cells, as LM-511 promotes cell migration. In fact, the $\alpha6\beta1$ integrin, a receptor for LM-511, is upregulated in many cancers including breast, liver, melanoma, and non-small cell lung carcinoma (47). In this way, too, CAMs that promote more transitory interactions may be expressed, in order to facilitate rapid movement upon the ECM proteins, rather than stable, more permanent interactions (such as hemidesmosomes). Disregulated $\alpha6\beta4$ integrin expression is seen in prostate, breast, melanoma, and colon (47). $\alpha6\beta4$ integrin is responsible for formation of hemidesmosome structures with LM-332, which is a stable interaction of the cell with the matrix that prevents migration. By downregulating this integrin, cancer cells switch to a more migratory phenotype. In this way, cancer cells take cues from the environment, and utilize them for increased growth and migration.

6. REGULATION OF PROTEOLYTIC ENZYMES DURING CANCER PROGRESSION

In response to the extracellular environment, another event that occurs is an increase of proteolytic enzymes in cancer cells. These proteolytic enzymes are important for the remodeling of the extracellular matrix in normal tissue. The most extensively studied proteolytic enzymes are the metalloproteases. There are two closely related metalloprotease families: MMPs and metalloprotease-disintegrins (ADAMs). MMPs are a family of over 20 enzymes that are characterized by their activity at neutral pH, ability to degrade the ECM, and their dependence on Zn^{2+} binding for proteolytic activity (48, 49). ADAMs are transmembrane proteins that contain disintegrin and metalloprotease domains, indicative of cell adhesion and protease activities (50). Studies have provided compelling evidence that MMP activity can induce or enhance tumor growth, survival, invasion, angiogenesis, and metastasis, whereas ADAM function is more focused, regulating growth signaling and tumor cell adhesion. These proteolytic enzymes play an important role in normal processes such as wound healing, vasculogenesis, axon outgrowth, and joint remodeling (51, 52). In wound healing, degradation of the ECM allows cells to enter the wounded site to repair (fill-in) that damage (53).

Cancer cells upregulate proteolytic enzymes in order to break down surrounding ECM which forms a barrier to migration. By degrading ECM proteins, cancer cells are no longer held back by a barrier of proteins, and are free to migrate through holes in the matrix. This is especially well-documented for cleavage of fibronectin by MMP-2, which leads to increased migration and proliferation of cells (54). However, proteolytic enzymes do much more than simply create a pathway for migration.

6.1 Release of Growth Factors

ECM proteins sequester growth factors within the matrix. Binding proteins like growth factors and cytokines is an important process because it stockpiles proteins that cells need in order to survive, and keeps a continual supply present. When ECM proteins are cleaved by proteolytic enzymes, these growth factors and other proteins are released from their interactions with the ECM proteins, and can bind to growth factor receptors on the cell surface. This, in turn, initiates new signaling pathways that can regulate growth and migration as well. By degrading ECM proteins, cancer cells release factors that induce growth and invasion. Because of the negative charge and varying pore sizes of glycosoaminoglycans and the GAG-chains of proteoglycans these molecules can act as a molecular sieve which controls the storage and traffic of signaling molecules according to their size and charge (55).

Stromelysin cleavage of ECM proteins releases various growth factors (56). The growth factors, epidermal growth factor (EGF) and acidic and basic fibroblast growth factors (aFGFs and bFGFs), which affect proliferation of many cell types, can be stored in heparin-sulphate chains of extracellular proteoglycans and may be released by heparinases during tumor invasion (55, 57, 58). Heparinase expressed by platelets, tumor, and inflammatory cells can release an active heparan sulfate-bound form of FGF-2 from the ECM (59). Cleavage of decorin by MMPs -2, -3, and -7 releases bound TGF-β1 (60). In addition to releasing TGF-β, MMPs can also activate latent TGF-β, as well as other latent growth factors in the extracellular environment. MMP-9 and MMP-2 can proteolytically cleave latent TGF-β *in vitro,* providing a novel mechanism for TGF-β activation (49). In addition, cytokines such as EGF, bFGF, and tumor necrosis factor-α (TNF-α) can stimulate transcription of several MMP genes (61-63).

6.2 Release of Growth Factor-Like Protein Fragments

Finally, when proteolytic enzymes break down ECM proteins, they cause the fragmentation of ECM proteins. ECM proteins contain structural and functional domains. These domains recognize cell surface receptors or other components of ECM. It is through these domains that ECM proteins form their highly organized three-dimensional matrix in which the proteins associate with each other and with cells. ECM proteins contain amino acid sequences for domains that not only bind to CAM receptors (adhesion receptor ligands), but also contain cryptic domains with structures similar to growth factors and cytokines. Fragments of ECM that are released containing these domains are called matrikines because they are basically cytokines that form from the matrix or are a part of intact matrix proteins (64).

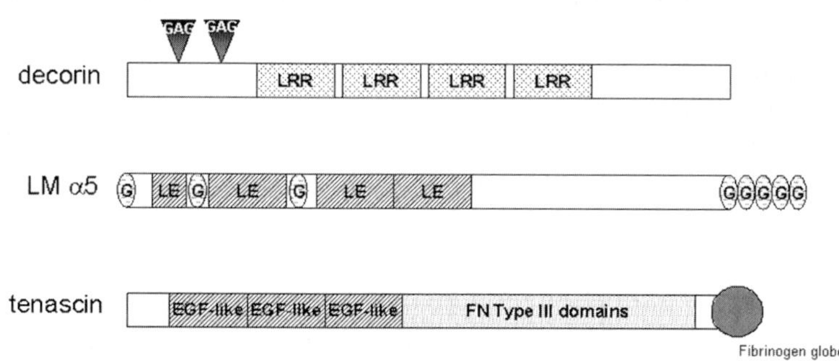

Figure 2. Cryptic domains within ECM proteins. Structural representation of ECM proteins and domains within the proteins that may be cleaved by proteases and function as matrikines. Decorin has Leucine-rich repeats (LRR) that can bind EGFR. Also indicated are GAG attachment sites (GAG). LM α5 chain has EGF-like repeats (LE) that may be solubilized upon cleavage with MT1-MMP. Also indicated are LM globular domains (G). Tenascin includes EGF-like repeats (EGF-like) and FN Type III domains.

Matrikine effects on cancer cells are the same as growth factors that are released from interactions with the ECM in that they can bind to growth factor receptors to initiate new signaling cascades. Commonly occurring matrikines in ECM proteins include EGF-like repeats of tenascin-C and laminin, and the leucine-rich region of decorin (LRR) modeled in Figure 2, which bind established receptor tyrosine kinases (65-67). Rat LM-332 is cleaved by MMP-2 which releases a fragment promoting cell migration (68). The LM-332 γ2 chain can also be cleaved by other proteases, causing enhanced cell migration on cleaved LM-332. Fragments of the γ2 chain can be detected in circulation (44). In addition, γ1 chain fragments of LM-α1β1γ1 (LM-111) have been observed in human circulation of cancer patients (69). The approximately 50 kDa N-terminal globular domains of γ1 and γ2 have been shown to possess EGF-like activity and bind the EGFR (70, 71) and γ2 can activate ERK1/2 phosphorylation. We have shown that human LM-332 β2 chain is cleaved by MT1-MMP and this fragment also has functional effects on migration (72). In prostate cancer, since LM-332 is not expressed, we propose the LM-332 cleavage is important for the progression of normal prostate to PIN, where LM-332 expression remains, and MT1-MMP is upregulated. In invasive prostate cancer, the surrounding BL consists mainly of LM-511, and we have also shown the LM-511 α5 chain is cleaved by MT1-MMP, releasing a soluble 45 kDa N-terminal fragment (73). This fragment contains EGF-like repeats similarly to the γ1 and γ2 fragments, and we propose that this α5 fragment functions similarly in invasive prostate cancer. Cryptic matrikines include short peptide sequences rather than structural repeats, such as IV-HL (GVKGDKGNPGWPGAP) from the major triple helical domain of the α1 chain of collagen IV (74). These peptide sequences tend to bind integrins as their receptors, but with unique signaling properties (75). Interestingly, unlike typical growth factors from the EGF family, the EGF-like repeats of tenascin-C and LM-332 signal to various cells in a distinctly pro-migratory fashion without evidence of significant proliferation (71, 76).

7. BASIC PROCESS OF METASTASIS

Taken together, the changing ECM ligands during cancer progression all function to make cancer cells more likely to succeed as they attempt to metastasize. Laying down a new basement membrane allows cancer cells to coordinate cellular events to take advantage of their new surrounding, be that for increased growth or increased migration. Changing ECM protein expression also allows for the upregulation of CAMs that will initiate more transitory cell adhesion to the new matrix, thereby promoting a more migratory cell phenotype on a matrix associated with migration. Upregulating proteolytic enzymes not only creates a pathway for migration, but puts the cancer cell in direct interaction with growth factors and matrikines released by or formed from ECM proteins to again promote growth and migration.

In order for a cancer cell to metastasize, it must first break through the ECM barrier to migration. It does this through upregulation of proteolytic enzymes, and by breaking down ECM proteins, it stimulates growth and invasion with factors released due to ECM protein degradation. Cancer cells migrate out of their initial site of growth toward a blood vessel or nerve to migrate to a different part of the body through the bloodstream. Following a growth factor trail in the ECM is one way in which the cancer cells succeed in doing this. Once in the bloodstream, the cancer cell must survive, and eventually extravasate out into a new site (77-80). CAMs that are expressed by the cancer cells help with this extravasation and fragments of ECM proteins can promote survival in the bloodstream, as can interactions with other cells through tight cell-cell adhesions. By being able to secrete their own matrix proteins, cancer cells that extravasate into new tissue ensure their survival by providing their own physical support system for growth until they are established. Degraded ECM components can then trigger further induction of protease genes, resulting in a positive feedback loop that further facilitates invasion and proliferation. The release of growth factors upon degradation of the ECM also facilitates tumor cell growth.

Similar mechanisms are shared by physiological and neoplastic invasion. In either case, the rate-limiting step for metastasis is the breakdown of connective tissue barriers (ECM) comprising collagens, laminins, fibronectin, vitronectin, and heparin sulfate proteoglycans, which requires the action of MMPs. The difference between them is that physiological invasion is regulated, whereas tumorigenesis invasion appears to be perpetual.

8. CONCLUDING REMARKS

In this chapter, we have described how the changing extracellular environment affects cancer metastasis. Events that at first appear uncoordinated (proteolysis and changing protein expression) actually function synergistically to enhance the metastatic process. These alterations and their effects on migration are represented in Figure 3. Altered ECM proteins cause altered CAM expression and signaling, which upregulates proteolytic enzymes. Altered ECM proteins signal for increased migration and proteolytic enzymes degrade matrix to enhance the migration.

Proteolytic cleavage of the ECM releases growth factors or matrikines, which enhance the signaling for migration as well as for expression of more proteolytic enzymes. For metastasis to be successful, these inter-related processes must all occur because these processes are typical of a cancer cell evading normal growth or migration control mechanisms through a disregulation of that controlled system. Although the actual coordination of metastatic events is unknown, changes in ECM ligands play an important role in the process.

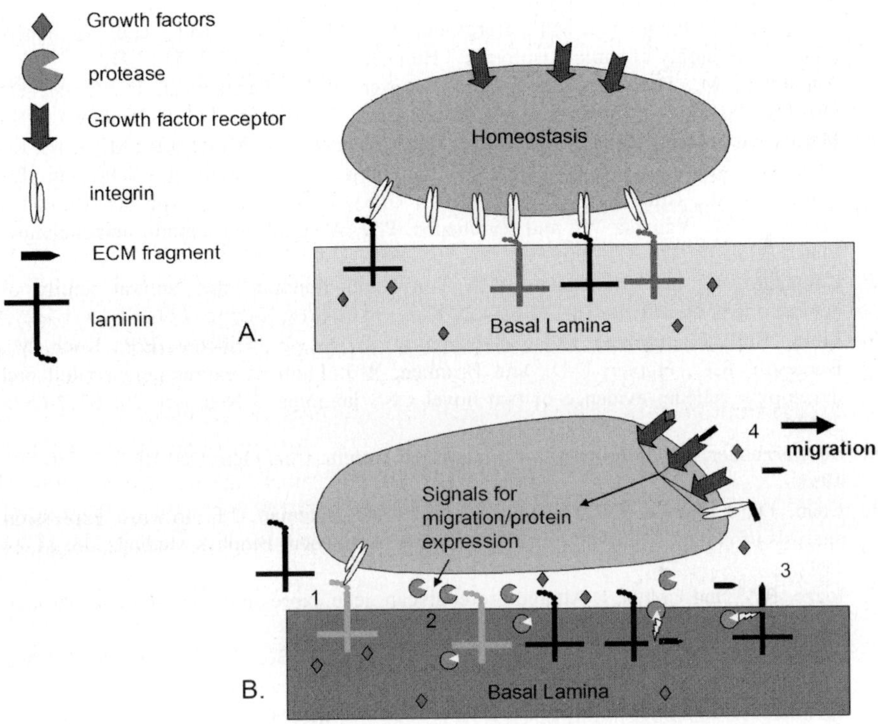

Figure 3. Changes in the extracellular environment that effect migration. A) A normal cell in homeostasis with regulated integrin adhesion, ECM protein expression and growth factor receptor function. B) A transformed cell that 1) secretes new ECM proteins altering the basal lamina, and 2) secreted proteolytic enzymes that 3) cleave ECM proteins such as laminins releasing matrikines and growth factors from the ECM that 4) interact with growth factor receptors and/or integrins to signal for cell migration.

REFERENCES

1. Timpl, R. and Aumailley, M. Biochemistry of basement membranes. Adv Nephrol Necker Hosp, 18: 59-76, 1989.
2. Erickson, A.C. and Couchman, J.R. Still more complexity in mammalian basement membranes. J Histochem Cytochem, 48: 1291-1306 2000.
3. Timpl, R. and Brown, J.C. Supramolecular assembly of basement membranes. Bioessays, 18: 123-132 1996.
4. Timpl, R., Macromolecular organization of basement membranes. Curr Opin Cell Biol, 8: 618-624 1996.
5. Yurchenco, P.D. and O'Rear, J.J. Basal lamina assembly. Curr Opin Cell Biol, 6: 674-681 1994.
6. Cheng, Y.S., Champliaud, M.F., Burgeson, R.E., Marinkovich, M.P., and Yurchenco, P.D. Self-assembly of laminin isoforms. J Biol Chem, 272: 31525-31532 1997.
7. Aumailley, M., Bruckner-Tuderman, L., Carter, W.G., Deutzmann, R., Edgar, D., Ekblom, P., Engel, J., Engvall, E., Hohenester, E., Jones, J.C., Kleinman, H.K., Marinkovich, M.P., Martin, G.R., Mayer, U., Meneguzzi, G., Miner, J.H., Miyazaki, K., Patarroyo, M., Paulsson, M., Quaranta, V., Sanes, J.R., Sasaki, T., Sekiguchi, K., Sorokin, L.M., Talts, J.F., Tryggvason, K., Uitto, J., Virtanen, I., von der Mark, K., Wewer, U.M., Yamada, Y., and Yurchenco, P.D. A simplified laminin nomenclature. Matrix Biol, 24: 326-332 2005.
8. Colognato, H. and Yurchenco, P.D. Form and function: the laminin family of heterotrimers. Dev Dyn, 218: 213-234 2000.
9. Libby, R.T., Champliaud, M.F., Claudepierre, T., Xu, Y., Gibbons, E.P., Koch, M., Burgeson, R.E., Hunter, D.D., and Brunken, W.J. Laminin expression in adult and developing retinae: evidence of two novel CNS laminins. J Neurosci, 20: 6517-6528 2000.
10. Schwarzbauer, J.E., Fibronectin: from gene to protein. Curr Opin Cell Biol, 3: 786-791 1991.
11. Chan, D., Lamande, S.R., McQuillan, D.J., and Bateman, J.F. In vitro expression analysis of collagen biosynthesis and assembly. J Biochem Biophys Methods, 36: 11-29 1997.
12. Iozzo, R.V. and Cohen, I. Altered proteoglycan gene expression and the tumor stroma. Experientia, 49: 447-455 1993.
13. Aberdam, D., Galliano, M.F., Vailly, J., Pulkkinen, L., Bonifas, J., Christiano, A.M., Tryggvason, K., Uitto, J., Epstein, E.H., Ortonne, J.P. Jr., and et al., Herlitz's junctional epidermolysis bullosa is linked to mutations in the gene (LAMC2) for the gamma 2 subunit of nicein/kalinin (LAMININ-5). Nat Genet, 6: 299-304 1994.
14. Nakano, A., Pfendner, E., Hashimoto, I., and Uitto, J. Herlitz junctional epidermolysis bullosa: novel and recurrent mutations in the LAMB3 gene and the population carrier frequency. J Invest Dermatol, 115: 493-498 2000.
15. Pulkkinen, L., Gerecke, D.R., Christiano, A.M., Wagman, D.W., Burgeson, R.E., and Uitto, J. Cloning of the beta 3 chain gene (LAMB3) of human laminin 5, a candidate gene in junctional epidermolysis bullosa. Genomics, 25: 192-198 1995.
16. Schwartz, M.A., Schaller, M.D., and Ginsberg, M.H., Integrins: emerging paradigms of signal transduction. Annu Rev Cell Dev Biol, 11: 549-599 1995.
17. Wary, K.K., Mariotti, A., Zurzolo, C., and Giancotti, F.G. A requirement for caveolin-1 and associated kinase Fyn in integrin signaling and anchorage-dependent cell growth. Cell, 94: 625-634 1998.

18. Clark, E.A. and Brugge, J.S. Integrins and signal transduction pathways: the road taken. Science, 268: 233-239 1995.
19. Giancotti, F.G. and Ruoslahti, E. Integrin signaling. Science, 285: 1028-1032 1999.
20. LaFlamme, S.E. and Auer, K.L. Integrin signaling. Semin Cancer Biol, 7: 111-118 1996.
21. Frisch, S.M. and Ruoslahti, E. Integrins and anoikis. Curr Opin Cell Biol, 9: 701-706 1997.
22. Barcellos-Hoff, M.H., Aggeler, J., Ram, T.G., and Bissell, M.J. Functional differentiation and alveolar morphogenesis of primary mammary cultures on reconstituted basement membrane. Development, 105: 223-235 1989.
23. Gumbiner, B.M., Cell adhesion: the molecular basis of tissue architecture and morphogenesis. Cell, 84: 345-357 1996.
24. Carey, D.J., Todd, M.S., and Rafferty, C.M. Schwann cell myelination: induction by exogenous basement membrane-like extracellular matrix. J Cell Biol, 102: 2254-2263 1986.
25. Bissell, D.M., Arenson, D.M., Maher, J.J., and Roll, F.J. Support of cultured hepatocytes by a laminin-rich gel. Evidence for a functionally significant subendothelial matrix in normal rat liver. J Clin Invest, 79: 801-812 1987.
26. Schuetz, E.G., Li, D., Omiecinski, C.J., Muller-Eberhard, U., Kleinman, H.K., Elswick, B., and Guzelian, P.S. Regulation of gene expression in adult rat hepatocytes cultured on a basement membrane matrix. J Cell Physiol, 134: 309-323 1988.
27. Kubota, Y., Kleinman, H.K., Martin, G.R., and Lawley, T.J. Role of laminin and basement membrane in the morphological differentiation of human endothelial cells into capillary-like structures. J Cell Biol, 107: 1589-1598 1988.
28. Tenniswood, M.P., Guenette, R.S., Lakins, J., Mooibroek, M., Wong, P., and Welsh, J.E. Active cell death in hormone-dependent tissues. Cancer Metastasis Rev, 11: 197-220 1992.
29. Lochter, A. and Bissell, M.J. An odyssey from breast to bone: multi-step control of mammary metastases and osteolysis by matrix metalloproteinases. Apmis, 107: 128-136 1999.
30. Cress, A.E., Rabinovitz, I., Zhu, W., and Nagle, R.B. The alpha 6 beta 1 and alpha 6 beta 4 integrins in human prostate cancer progression. Cancer Metastasis Rev, 14: 219-228 1995.
31. Tani, T., Karttunen, T., Kiviluoto, T., Kivilaakso, E., Burgeson, R.E., Sipponen, P., and Virtanen, I. Alpha 6 beta 4 integrin and newly deposited laminin-1 and laminin-5 form the adhesion mechanism of gastric carcinoma. Continuous expression of laminins but not that of collagen VII is preserved in invasive parts of the carcinomas: implications for acquisition of the invading phenotype. Am J Pathol, 149: 781-793 1996.
32. Nagle, R.B., Knox, J.D., Wolf, C., Bowden, G.T., and Cress, A.E. Adhesion molecules, extracellular matrix, and proteases in prostate carcinoma. J Cell Biochem Suppl, 19: 232-237 1994.
33. Horgan, K., Jones, D.L., and Mansel, R.E. Mitogenicity of human fibroblasts *in vivo* for human breast cancer cells. Br J Surg, 74: 227-229 1987.
34. Ronnov-Jessen, L. and Petersen, O.W. Induction of alpha-smooth muscle actin by transforming growth factor-beta 1 in quiescent human breast gland fibroblasts. Implications for myofibroblast generation in breast neoplasia. Lab Invest, 68: 696-707 1993.
35. Ellis, M.J., Singer, C., Hornby, A., Rasmussen, A., and Cullen, K.J. Insulin-like growth factor mediated stromal-epithelial interactions in human breast cancer. Breast Cancer Res Treat, 31: 249-261 1994.

36. Bronzert, D.A., Pantazis, P., Antoniades, H.N., Kasid, A., Davidson, N., Dickson, R.B., and Lippman, M.E. Synthesis and secretion of platelet-derived growth factor by human breast cancer cell lines. Proc Natl Acad Sci U S A, 84: 5763-5767 1987.
37. Shao, Z.M., Nguyen, M., and Barsky, S.H. Human breast carcinoma desmoplasia is PDGF initiated. Oncogene, 19: 4337-4345 2000.
38. Ziober, B.L., Lin, C.S., and Kramer, R.H. Laminin-binding integrins in tumor progression and metastasis. Semin Cancer Biol, 7: 119-128 1996.
39. Peters, B.P., Hartle, R.J., Krzesicki, R.F., Kroll, T.G., Perini, F., Balun, J.E., Goldstein, I.J., and Ruddon, R.W. The biosynthesis, processing, and secretion of laminin by human choriocarcinoma cells. J Biol Chem, 260: 14732-14742 1985.
40. Frenette, G.P., Carey, T.E., Varani, J., Schwartz, D.R., Fligiel, S.E., Ruddon, R.W., and Peters, B.P. Biosynthesis and secretion of laminin and laminin-associated glycoproteins by nonmalignant and malignant human keratinocytes: comparison of cell lines from primary and secondary tumors in the same patient. Cancer Res, 48: 5193-5202 1988.
41. Pyke, C., Romer, J., Kallunki, P., Lund, L.R., Ralfkiaer, E., Dano, K., and Tryggvason, K. The gamma 2 chain of kalinin/laminin 5 is preferentially expressed in invading malignant cells in human cancers. Am J Pathol, 145: 782-791 1994.
42. Akiyama, S.K., Olden, K., and Yamada, K.M. Fibronectin and integrins in invasion and metastasis. Cancer Metastasis Rev, 14: 173-189 1995.
43. Hao, J., Yang, Y. McDaniel, K.M., Dalkin, B.L., Cress, A.E., and Nagle, R.B. Differential expression of laminin 5 (alpha 3 beta 3 gamma 2) by human malignant and normal prostate. Am J Pathol, 149: 1341-1349 1996.
44. Katayama, M., Sanzen, N., Funakoshi, A., and Sekiguchi, K. Laminin gamma2-chain fragment in the circulation: a prognostic indicator of epithelial tumor invasion. Cancer Res, 63: 222-229 2003.
45. Takeichi, M., Cadherin cell adhesion receptors as a morphogenetic regulator. Science, 251: 1451-1455 1991.
46. Ruoslahti, E., The Walter Herbert Lecture. Control of cell motility and tumour invasion by extracellular matrix interactions. Br J Cancer, 66: 239-242 1992.
47. Mizejewski, G.J., Role of integrins in cancer: survey of expression patterns. Proc Soc Exp Biol Med, 222: 124-138 1999.
48. Westermarck, J. and Kahari, V.M. Regulation of matrix metalloproteinase expression in tumor invasion. FASEB J, 13: 781-792 1999.
49. Yu, Q. and Stamenkovic, I. Cell surface-localized matrix metalloproteinase-9 proteolytically activates TGF-beta and promotes tumor invasion and angiogenesis. Genes Dev, 14: 163-176 2000.
50. Primakoff, P. and Myles, D.G. The ADAM gene family: surface proteins with adhesion and protease activity. Trends Genet, 16: 83-87 2000.
51. Holmbeck, K., Bianco, P., Caterina, J., Yamada, S., Kromer, M., Kuznetsov, S.A., Mankani, M., Robey, P.G., Poole, A.R., Pidoux, I., Ward, J.M., and Birkedal-Hansen, H. MT1-MMP-deficient mice develop dwarfism, osteopenia, arthritis, and connective tissue disease due to inadequate collagen turnover. Cell, 99: 81-92 1999.
52. Bullard, K.M., Lund, L., Mudgett, J.S., Mellin, T.N., Hunt, T.K., Murphy, B., Ronan, J., Werb, Z., and Banda, M.J. Impaired wound contraction in stromelysin-1-deficient mice. Ann Surg, 230: 260-265 1999.
53. Beare, A.H., O'Kane, S., Krane, S.M., and Ferguson, M.W. Severely impaired wound healing in the collagenase-resistant mouse. J Invest Dermatol, 120: 153-163 2003.
54. Grant, M.B., Caballero, S., Bush, D.M., and Spoerri, P.E. Fibronectin fragments modulate human retinal capillary cell proliferation and migration. Diabetes, 47: 1335-1340 1998.

55. Ruoslahti, E. and Yamaguchi, Y. Proteoglycans as modulators of growth factor activities. Cell, 64: 867-869 1991.
56. Masson, R., Lefebvre, O., Noel, A., Fahime, M.E., Chenard, M.P., Wendling, C., Kebers, F., LeMeur, M., Dierich, A., Foidart, J.M., Basset, P., and Rio, M.C. In vivo evidence that the stromelysin-3 metalloproteinase contributes in a paracrine manner to epithelial cell malignancy. J Cell Biol, 140: 1535-1541 1998.
57. Flaumenhaft, R., Moscatelli, D., and Rifkin, D.B. Heparin and heparan sulfate increase the radius of diffusion and action of basic fibroblast growth factor. J Cell Biol, 111: 1651-1659 1990.
58. Vlodavsky, I., Bar-Shavit, R., Ishai-Michaeli, R., Bashkin, P., and Fuks, Z. Extracellular sequestration and release of fibroblast growth factor: a regulatory mechanism? Trends Biochem Sci, 16: 268-271 1991.
59. Vlodavsky, I. and Friedmann, Y. Molecular properties and involvement of heparanase in cancer metastasis and angiogenesis. J Clin Invest, 108: 341-347 2001.
60. Imai, K., Hiramatsu, A., Fukushima, D., Pierschbacher, M.D., and Okada, Y. Degradation of decorin by matrix metalloproteinases: identification of the cleavage sites, kinetic analyses and transforming growth factor-beta1 release. Biochem J, 322 (Pt 3): 809-814 1997.
61. Gavrilovic, J., Moens, G., Thiery, J.P., and Jouanneau, J. Expression of transfected transforming growth factor alpha induces a motile fibroblast-like phenotype with extracellular matrix-degrading potential in a rat bladder carcinoma cell line. Cell Regul, 1: 1003-1014 1990.
62. Jouanneau, J., Gavrilovic, J., Caruelle, D., Jaye, M., Moens, G., Caruelle, J.P., and Thiery, J.P. Secreted or nonsecreted forms of acidic fibroblast growth factor produced by transfected epithelial cells influence cell morphology, motility, and invasive potential. Proc Natl Acad Sci U S A, 88: 2893-2897 1991.
63. Wernert, N., Gilles, F., Fafeur, V., Bouali, F., Raes, M.B., Pyke, C., Dupressoir, T., Seitz, G., Vandenbunder, B., and Stehelin, D. Stromal expression of c-Ets1 transcription factor correlates with tumor invasion. Cancer Res, 54: 5683-5688 1994.
64. Maquart, F.X., Simeon, A., Pasco, S., and Monboisse, J.C. [Regulation of cell activity by the extracellular matrix: the concept of matrikines]. J Soc Biol, 193: 423-428 1999.
65. Swindle, C.S., Tran, K.T., Johnson, T.D., Banerjee, P., Mayes, A.M., Griffith, L., and Wells, A. Epidermal growth factor (EGF)-like repeats of human tenascin-C as ligands for EGF receptor. J Cell Biol, 154: 459-468 2001.
66. Shrivastava, A., Radziejewski, C., Campbell, E., Kovac, L., McGlynn, M., Ryan, T.E., Davis, S., Goldfarb, M.P., Glass, D.J., Lemke, G., and Yancopoulos, G.D. An orphan receptor tyrosine kinase family whose members serve as nonintegrin collagen receptors. Mol Cell, 1: 25-34 1997.
67. Santra, M., Reed, C.C., and Iozzo, R.V. Decorin binds to a narrow region of the epidermal growth factor (EGF) receptor, partially overlapping but distinct from the EGF-binding epitope. J Biol Chem, 277: 35671-35681 2002.
68. Giannelli, G., Falk-Marzillier, J., Schiraldi, O., Stetler-Stevenson, W.G., and Quaranta, V. Induction of cell migration by matrix metalloprotease-2 cleavage of laminin-5. Science, 277: 225-228 1997.
69. Byers, L.J., Osborne, J.L., Carson, L.F., Carter, J.R., Haney, A.F., Weinberg, J.B., and Ramakrishnan, S. Increased levels of laminin in ascitic fluid of patients with ovarian cancer. Cancer Lett, 88: 67-72 1995.
70. Panayotou, G., End, P., Aumailley, M., Timpl, R., and Engel, J. Domains of laminin with growth-factor activity. Cell, 56: 93-101 1989.

71. Schenk, S., Hintermann, E., Bilban, M., Koshikawa, N., Hojilla, C., Khokha, R., and Quaranta, V. Binding to EGF receptor of a laminin-5 EGF-like fragment liberated during MMP-dependent mammary gland involution. J Cell Biol, 161: 197-209 2003.
72. Udayakumar, T.S., Chen, M.L., Bair, E.L., Von Bredow, D.C., Cress, A.E., Nagle, R.B., and Bowden, G.T. Membrane type-1-matrix metalloproteinase expressed by prostate carcinoma cells cleaves human laminin-5 beta3 chain and induces cell migration. Cancer Res, 63: 2292-2299 2003.
73. Bair, E.L., Chen, M.L., McDaniel, K., Sekiguchi, K., Cress, A.E., Nagle, R.B., and Bowden, G.T. Membrane type 1 matrix metalloprotease cleaves laminin-10 and promotes prostate cancer cell migration. Neoplasia, 7: 380-389 2005.
74. Chelberg, M.K., McCarthy, J.B., Skubitz, A.P., Furcht, L.T., and Tsilibary E.C. Characterization of a synthetic peptide from type IV collagen that promotes melanoma cell adhesion, spreading, and motility. J Cell Biol, 111: 261-270 1990.
75. Sudhakar, A., Sugimoto, H., Yang, C., Lively, J., Zeisberg, M., and Kalluri, R. Human tumstatin and human endostatin exhibit distinct antiangiogenic activities mediated by alpha v beta 3 and alpha 5 beta 1 integrins. Proc Natl Acad Sci U S A, 100: 4766-4771 2003.
76. Schenk, S. and Quaranta, V. Tales from the crypt[ic] sites of the extracellular matrix. Trends Cell Biol, 13: 366-375 2003.
77. Folkman, J. The role of angiogenesis in tumor growth. Semin Cancer Biol, 3: 65-71 1992.
78. Woodhouse, E.C., Chuaqui, R.F., and Liotta, L.A. General mechanisms of metastasis. Cancer, 80: 1529-1537 1997.
79. Fidler, I.J., Critical determinants of cancer metastasis: rationale for therapy. Cancer Chemother Pharmacol, 43 Suppl: S3-10 1999.
80. Chambers, A.F., Naumov, G.N., Varghese, H.J., Nadkarni, K.V., MacDonald, I.C., and Groom, A.C. Critical steps in hematogenous metastasis: an overview. Surg Oncol Clin N Am, 10: 243-255, 2001.

Chapter 2

SUPPRESSION AND ALTERATION OF ADHESION STRUCTURES IN HUMAN EPITHELIAL CANCER PROGRESSION

Tracy L. Davis[1], Aaron J. Goldman[2] and Anne E. Cress[3]
[1]Department of Pathology, Massachusetts General Hospital, Boston, Massachusetts, USA
[2]Department of Molecular and Cellular Biology, University of Arizona, Tucson, Arizona, USA
[3]Department of Cell Biology and Anatomy, University of Arizona, Tucson, Arizona, USA

Abstract: An early step in epithelial cancer progression is the loss of cell adhesion structures and the persistence of selected sets of adhesion proteins. In this chapter, the data from immunohistochemical analysis of human tissue and published DNA microarray results from human tissue are discussed to illustrate the altered expression of cell adhesion structures in carcinomas. Further, the role of adhesion structures in cancer metastasis is discussed and the inherited alterations in adhesion molecules associated with increased risk for certain carcinomas is detailed. Finally, the potential utility of elements of the adhesion structures as surrogate and end point biomarkers is discussed.

Key words: adhesion; carcinoma; extracellular matrix; hemidesmosome; cytokeratin; laminin; CD151; integrin; prostate cancer; colon cancer; breast cancer

1. INTRODUCTION

Cell adhesion is responsible for the three-dimensional organization, stability and viability of tissue in mammals. Through extracellular protein interactions as well as intracellular and anchoring motifs, cell adhesions provide a construct for many necessary interactions. Communicating junctions such as gap junctions, anchoring junctions such as desmosomes and adherens junctions, and sealing junctions such as zonula occludens or tight junctions all provide the robust scaffold for epithelial architecture. It is this construction of the anchoring of cells to the basement membrane that is the most crucial for the function and integrity of various tissues. Epithelial

A.E. Cress and R.B. Nagle (eds.), Cell Adhesion and Cytoskeletal Molecules in Metastasis, 19–46.

cell adhesion is achieved by maintaining a unique composition of proteins at the basal side facing the extracellular matrix and at the apical side facing the lumen.

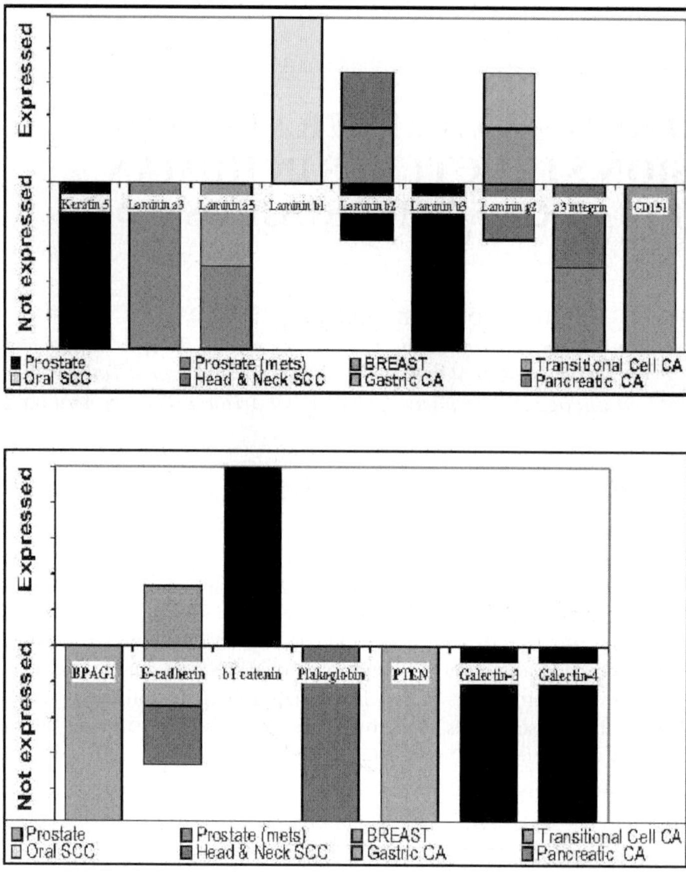

Figure 1. Suppression of Adhesion Related Proteins in Human Cancer Tissues. The expression status of selected known adhesion related proteins is derived from published reports cited in the text using immunohistochemistry based estimates of protein expression.
Top panel: Cytokeratin 5 (keratin 5), Laminin alpha 3 chain (laminin a3), Laminin alpha 5 chain (laminin a5), Laminin beta1 chain (laminin b1), Laminin beta2 chain (laminin b2), Laminin beta3 chain (laminin b3), Laminin gamma3 chain (Laminin G3), alpha3 Integrin (a3 Integrin) and CD151 (CD151) were scored within the tissues as indicated by the corresponding patterned bars.
Bottom Panel: Bullous Pemphigoid Antigen (BPAG1), E-cadherin (E-cadherin), beta1 catenin (b1 catentin), Plakoglobin (plakoglobin), Phosphatase and Tensin Homolog (PTEN) and Galectin 3 and Galectin 4 were scored within the selected tissues as indicated by the corresponding patterned bars.

Loss or alteration of adhesion structures in epithelial tumors is a well-known phenomenon that commonly occurs during tumor progression (Figure 1). Studies in prostate cancer progression have revealed dramatic loss of the hemidesmosome protein complex, which combined with dysregulated production of metalloproteases and pro-migratory signals, is thought to be important for cancer cell invasion and metastasis. Additionally, alteration of other cell adhesion structures (desmosomes, adherens junctions and tight junctions) has been shown to occur in prostate and many other epithelial tumors (Figure 2).

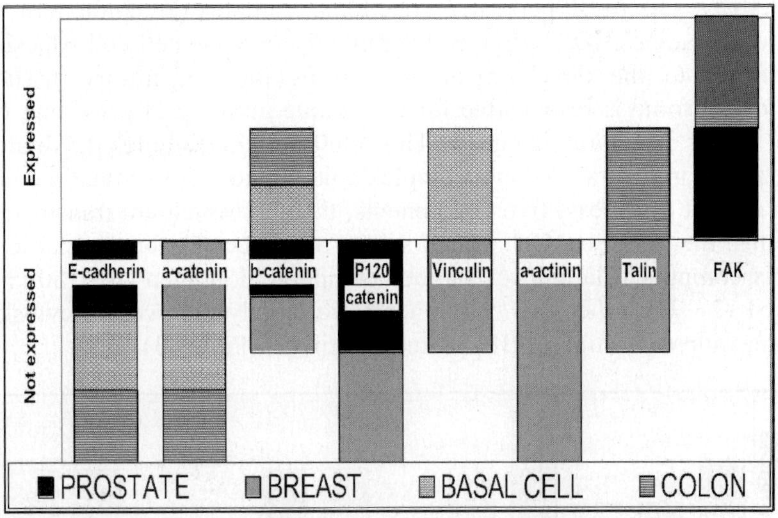

Figure 2. Suppression of Adherens Junction Type Proteins in Human Epithelial Cancers. The expression status of selected known adhesion related proteins is derived from published reports cited in the text. The graph illustrates whether the proteins are either expressed or not expressed as indicated by immunohistochemistry based estimates of protein expression. The selected tissues assayed are as indicated by the corresponding patterned bars.

The field of cell adhesion and cancer is large and ever-expanding. For this reason, a chapter on the subject cannot be all-inclusive. We have chosen to focus on research obtained from primary human carcinomas and to limit the discussion to primarily to prostate, breast, colon, basal cell, and non-cutaneous squamous cell carcinomas.

2. ALTERED EXPRESSION OF CELL ADHESION STRUCTURES IN CARCINOMAS

In the following sections, we will describe the reported alterations in proteins known to be involved in cell adhesion structures during cancer progression. The reported alterations detailed here are restricted to studies investigating the expression patterns in human tissue (1, 2).

2.1 Hemidesmosomes

Perhaps the most pervasive junctional complex in epithelium is the hemidesmosome (HD). While cell communication and cell-cell adhesion are significant to the development and proliferation of normal tissue, the hemidesmosome is responsible for the unique property of providing tissues with strong structural integrity. This multiprotein complex facilitates the firm adhesion of stratified and complex epithelia to the basement membrane. HDs consist of at least five components, three of which are transmembrane proteins: the integrin $\alpha 6\beta 4$, which serves as a receptor for the extracellular matrix component laminin-5, bullous pemphigoid antigen (BP)180 (1); and CD151 (2). The other two components are largely involved in cytoskeletal organization consisting of BP230 and plectin (3) (Figure 3).

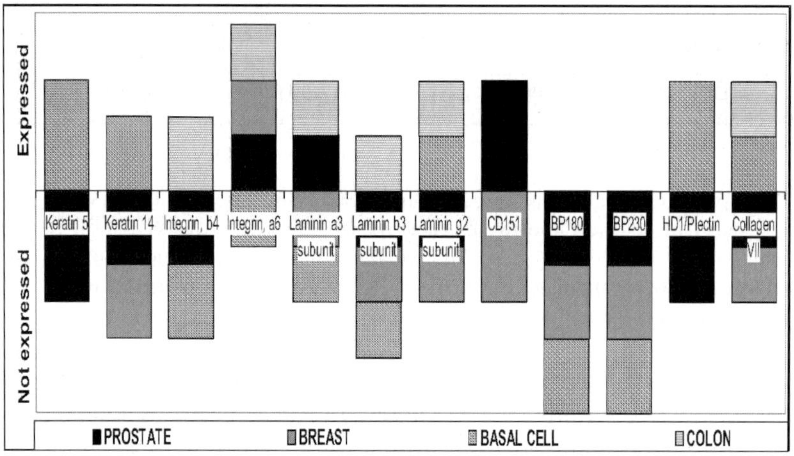

Figure 3. Microarray Expression Data On Hemidesmosomal Proteins Within Human Cancer Tissues. The mRNA expression status of selected known hemidesmosome related proteins was derived from published reports cited in the text. The graph illustrates whether the mRNA coding for the indicated twelve proteins are either expressed or not expressed as indicated DNA microarray data. The selected tissues assayed are as indicated by the corresponding patterned bars.

The hemidesmosome is a multiprotein complex assembled at the basal lamina of epithelial cells, which acts as an anchor between the intracellular cytokeratin network and the extracellular matrix. Hemidesmosomes play integral roles in maintaining normal tissue architecture. To date, at least eleven different proteins have been observed in hemidesmosomes, including integrins, (α6β4 integrin) cytokeratins (cytokeratin 5 and 14), extracellular matrix proteins (laminin-5, (332) consisting of α3, β3, γ2 subunits), bullous pemphigoid antigens (BP180 and BP230), IFAP300, LAD-1 plectin/HD1 and collagen VII. Selected examples of each of these proteins is discussed below.

2.2 α6β4 Integrin

The large variety of integrins mediate cell adhesion to the extracellular environment and are important for the integrity of cells by connecting the cytoskeleton to the plasma membrane (4). The α6β4 integrin is a significant intramembrane protein that defines the structural integrity of the hemidesmosome. At over 1000 amino acids long, the integrin β4 subunit is essential in the formation of the HD junctional complex (5). The hemidesmosome has largely and classically been implicated in rooting the architecture for cellular adhesion.

The α6β4 integrin is a transmembrane heterodimeric glycoprotein that is essential in hemidesmosome assembly which facilitates linkage between the cytoskeleton and the extracellular collagen VII network and is important for maintaining tissue architecture.

The α6β4 integrin has frequently been implicated in epithelial tumor progression, both positively and negatively. We propose loss of the α6β4 integrin, and resulting loss of the hemidesmosome, is important for enabling tumor cell migration and metastasis. Our studies of invasive prostate carcinoma have demonstrated loss of the α6β4 integrin (6-9), and other groups have also confirmed these findings (10-11). However expression of the α6 integrin in prostate carcinoma is maintained or even upregulated (7, 12). Furthermore, alterations in the α6β4 integrin are evident in early, precancerous PIN lesions (13). This suggests that changes in cell adhesion occur prior to genetic alterations such as p53 and Rb mutations, thus highlighting a potential role of adhesion proteins as biomarkers in diagnosis.

Loss of the α6β4 integrin has been reported in human breast carcinomas (13, 14). In a study of 53 human invasive breast carcinomas, 80% demonstrated loss of expression of the α6β4 integrin by immunohistochemistry (15). Interestingly, 66% of the cases demonstrated non-linear immunostaining and diffuse cytoplasmic staining of the α6β4 integrin in the non-involved breast tissue of the same patients, suggesting an inherent 'field defect' may be present that could predispose a subset of patients to development of cancer.

Loss of expression of the α6β4 integrin has been reported in skin cancers, including basal cell carcinoma, squamous cell carcinoma and squamous cell carcinoma *in situ* accompanied by increased expression of metalloproteases (16-19). In some studies, cutaneous squamous cell carcinomas have been demonstrated to express increased amounts of α6β4 integrin at both the gene and protein levels (19-20). While other studies have reported loss of polarized expression of α6β4 integrin in SCC with increased protein turnover (21) and ultrastructural loss of hemidesmosomes by EM studies (19).

In oral squamous cell carcinomas, one study demonstrated altered localization (suprabasal and pericellular) of the α6β4 integrin which is normally polarized along the basal lamina (22). Altered cellular localization of the α6 integrin subunit was also apparent in dysplastic epithelial samples as well. Western blot analysis revealed increased expression of the α6 integrin, but only minimal retrieval of the β4 subunit, suggesting the ratio of the α6 to β4 integrin subunits is altered in oral squamous cell carcinomas (and possibly also in dysplastic epithelium). Therefore, lack of α6 integrin polarization may be an early event in tumor progression.

In serous ovarian carcinomas, progression occurs by exfoliation of cells from the surface of the ovary. Tumor nests have an irregular basement membrane and carcinoma cells that have lost contact with the membrane, demonstrated loss of α6β4 integrin expression (23). Additionally, examination of the ovarian carcinoma ascites cells, revealed significantly decreased expression of α6β4 integrin, further strengthening the idea that loss of α6β4 integrin-mediated adhesion in tumor cells is associated with tumor progression.

Not all epithelial tumors demonstrate loss of α6β4 integrin, however. Neoexpression of α6β4 integrin has been reported in thyroid tumors, for example (24). Retention of and/or increased expression of α6β4 integrin in many colon carcinomas has also been reported (13, 25-29) and implicated in tumor progression and metastasis (25, 28, 29). Yet some groups have demonstrated loss of α6β4 integrin expression with tumor invasion and progression (30). In 1992, Stallmach and others reported expression of α6β4 integrin was maintained in colorectal adenomas, but the transformation from benign to malignant neoplasms associated with infiltrative growth was characterized by diminished or lost expression of α6 and β4 subunit chains (31). Furthermore, the laminin-5 deposited in colon adenomas and carcinomas may serve as a ligand for α3β1 integrin as well, which is a more promigratory ligand (26), again suggesting that colorectal carcinomas progress through a different mechanism than that of prostate.

One possibility for the contradictory reports of α6β4 integrin in epithelial tumors may be explained by the corruption of components of the integrin complex to facilitate adhesion dependent migration without the formation of the hemidesmosome (see Chapter 4, this volume). Alternatively, the ability of the hemidesmosome to dynamically associate into different subtypes (type I and type II hemidesmosomes) or "cross-talk" to other adhesion structures and thus play roles in focal adhesion and cell migration are possible (32, 33). A second type of hemidesmosome has been identified in the colon, termed a type II hemidesmosome (34-36). In cells which lack BP230 and BP180, α6β4 integrin can still associate with HD1 and form a type II hemidesmosome. Studies suggest that type II hemidesmosomes behave in a different manner compared with the conventionally studied type I hemidesmosomes (27).

2.3 Laminin-5

Laminin-5 is a significant component of the hemidesmosome and its loss of function or truncated translation results in such diseases as junctional epidermolysis bullosa (37).

Laminin-5 is a heterotrimeric protein component of the basal lamina and hemidesmosome protein complex. It functions to link the hemidesmosome via the α6β4 integrin to the underlying connective tissue and type VII collagen (38). Our group and others have reported loss of assembled laminin-5 protein expression in prostate cancer (6, 10, 39, 40). Furthermore loss of assembled laminin-5 deposition was evident in precancerous PIN lesions, suggesting alteration of adhesion is an early event in prostate tumor progression (13). Additionally, microarray analysis has suggested the β3 subunit of laminin-5 is downregulated in human prostate carcinoma (41), although this was not confirmed by Northern analysis.

The expression of laminin-5 in human breast carcinomas appears to be more variable (13, 42). One microarray study suggested 32% of breast carcinomas examined showed upregulation of the γ2 subunit (43).

Decreased expression of laminin-5 in cutaneous squamous cell carcinomas (cSCC) and basal cell carcinomas (BCC) has been reported by immunohistochemistry and quantitative PCR reactions (17, 18). Interestingly, in laminin-5 negative tumors, a faint cytoplasmic immunostaining for the γ2 subunit was apparent in 12 basal cell carcinomas examined (16), suggesting aberrant expression of laminin-5 occurs. Chopra and others postulated that the decreased levels of basement membrane proteins in skin carcinomas may lead to structural instability and facilitate invasion (17).

We and others have demonstrated that colorectal carcinomas retain expression of laminin-5 in linear distribution surrounding invasive glands (13, 26). Furthermore, it has been reported that increased expression of laminin-5 in colorectal carcinomas was associated with increased invasiveness and metastatic liver lesions (44). These data suggest that the colorectal carcinomas may progress through a distinct mechanism compared to other epithelial carcinomas. In colon adenomas, laminin-5, laminin 10 and collagen VII are expressed in the basement membranes, however in carcinoma tissues, the basement membrane is composed primarily of laminin-5, especially at the invading edges (26). Immunohistochemistry reveals the α3 integrin is present in all adenomas and most carcinomas, often co-localized with laminin-5. Function blocking antibodies to α3 integrin, but not α6 integrin inhibited cell adhesion in cell culture experiments, suggesting that the interaction between α3β1 and laminin-5 is more important for cell adhesion in colon carcinoma than that of α6β4 integrin. Although it remains to be demonstrated whether this phenomenon is true *in vivo*.

2.4 BP Antigens (BP180, BP230)

The BP antigens (BP180, BP230) were first identified as autoimmune antigens in bullous pemphigoid disease, a skin disease which results in a mild blistering phenotype. BP180 is a transmembrane collagenous protein (45) that interacts with the cytoplasmic domain of β4 integrin and is involved in the recruitment of BP230 to the hemidesmosome complex (46, 47). Additionally, it can bind to α6 integrin (48, 49). BP230 is a cytoplasmic protein that belongs to the plakin protein family that localizes to the intermediate filament attachment sites of the epithelial cell (50, 51). Recently, the N-terminal domain of BP230 has been shown to interact with BP180 (47) during hemidesmosome assembly.

We reported loss of expression of BP180 occurred in prostate carcinomas. Additionally, only 30% of tumors examined retained expression of BP230 (6), suggesting loss of these proteins is common in prostate cancer progression. Microarray studies have also suggested decreased expression of BP230 occurs in prostate carcinoma (41). Decreased expression of BP180 and BP230 has been reported in breast carcinomas (52). To date there is no conclusive data that colon tumors express BP180, but one report suggests they repress its expression (53).

In cutaneous squamous cell and basal cell carcinomas, down-regulation of both BP180 and BP230 has been reported (17, 54), although one group has reported increased expression of BP180 in squamous cell carcinomas (55). Furthermore, increased expression of BP230 in cutaneous SCC has also been reported and was positively correlated with increased cell invasion (19). The finding that the hemidesmosome is ultrastructurally lost suggests that portions of the remaining protein complex may function altogether differently compared to other epithelial carcinomas.

2.5 Plectin/HD1

Plectin is approximately a 500 kD phosphoprotein that is expressed in epithelial cells and functions as a cytoskeletal linking protein in the hemidesmosome complex. Recent evidence demonstrates that plectin is recruited to the hemidesmosome by direct interaction with the β4 integrin cytoplasmic tail, which then functions to recruit BP180 into the protein complex (56).

Loss of the cytoskeletal linking protein HD1/plectin has been reported in invasive prostate carcinoma, with only 15% of cases examined retaining expression (6) and in solid basal cell carcinomas (16, 18). These findings are in contrast to reports in colon carcinoma. In cultured human colon carcinoma cells, expression of HD1/plectin was found to be polarized and co-localized with α6β4 integrin (27). To date, the expression of HD1/plectin in human colorectal carcinomas has not been completely examined.

2.6 Collagen VII

Type VII collagen is a homotrimer of three α1 subchains and is the major component of the anchoring fibrils in epithelia (57, 58) which is necessary for stable adhesion via the hemidesmosome of cells to the extracellular matrix.

Loss of collagen VII expression has been reported by us and others in invasive prostate carcinoma (6, 8, 10), which corresponds with the loss of expression of nearly all other hemidesmosome component proteins. Additionally, loss of collagen VII has been reported in colon carcinomas and invasive bladder carcinomas (26, 61). Interestingly, collagen VII appears to be retained in basal cell carcinomas, as demonstrated by immunohistochemistry (16).

2.7 Keratins 5 and 14

Keratins are a member of the intermediate filament family and form alpha helical coiled-coil dimers that associate laterally to form 10 nm filaments as part of the cytoskeleton network in all epithelial cells. The keratins are subdivided into two sequence types (I and II) that are typically co-expressed as pairs (56). Keratins 5 (type II) and 14 (type I) are members of a multigene family and are the primary keratins of the basal cells of stratified epithelium. Loss of expression of cytokeratin 5 and 14 has been reported in several epithelial cancers including prostate adenocarcinomas (63, 64). Expression of keratin 5 is reportedly decreased in prostate carcinomas at both the protein and mRNA levels (41, 65-67).

Interestingly the gene expression of KRT14 was attenuated in PIN lesions while keratin 14 protein expression was entirely lost. This finding underscores the importance of loss of cell adhesion and architecture is an early phenomenon in prostate cancer progression.

Variablitity of cytokeratin expression has been reported in breast carcinomas (68, 69). Additionally, retention of cytokeratins 5 and 14 has been reported in basal cell carcinomas (70).

2.8 Adherens Junctions

The adherens junction is a multiprotein complex assembled between epithelial cells into heterodimeric complexes. They consist of transmembrane cadherins (E-cadherin and/or P-cadherin in squamous epithelial cells) linked to plakoglobin or b-catenin, which links to catenins (a-catenin, b-catenin, p120 catenin) and ultimately to the actin cytoskeleton. Numerous alterations of adhesion structures (desmosomes, adherens junctions, tight junctions) have been reported in epithelial tumors (71-77). Selected examples of these proteins are discussed below.

2.8.1 Cadherin-Catenin Complex

Loss of E-cadherin function in human epithelial carcinomas has been well documented (78-82). Expression of E-cadherin is thought to serve as a suppressor of invasion and growth, thus its functional loss represents a step in tumor progression (83).

In prostate carcinoma, expression of E-cadherin (84), β-catenin and p120 catenin (85) is downregulated, and this expression correlates with increased tumor grade (73, 86). One report demonstrated an increase in α-catenin, but decreased expression of β-catenin in both prostate carcinoma and benign prostatic hypertrophy (87). In breast carcinomas, expression of the E-cadherin-catenin complex (including α- and β-catenins, and p120) is also frequently lost (88-91).

Reduced expression of E-cadherin, α-catenin and β-catenin has been reported in cutaneous basal cell carcinomas (92, 93) with increased nuclear accumulation of β-catenins as evidenced by immunohistochemistry (94, 95).

Similarly, in colon carcinomas, loss of E-cadherin and α-catenin expression has been reported (96-98) with a subsequent increase in nuclear expression of β-catenin (99, 100).

Loss of E-cadherin expression has been associated with upregulation of N-cadherin expression in many epithelial tumors. Suppression of the classical adherens junction structure in tumors resulting from functional loss of E-cadherin and catenins may be associated with tumor progression.

2.8.2 Desmosome

The desmosome functions as a cell-cell adhesion multi-protein structure complex in epithelial cells. It is composed of transmembrane proteins from the cadherin family (desmogleins, desmocollins) which interact with linking proteins (desmoplakin, and plakoglobin) to ultimately link up to the intermediate filament cytoskeleton.

The expression of the desmosome proteins has been less well studied in human epithelial tumors. No data is available for functional expression of desmoglein, desmocollin, desmoplakin or plakoglobin in human prostate carcinomas, however data from cell lines suggests that prostate cancer cells have reduced expression of plakoglobin (101).

Loss of heterozygosity for plakoglobin (as evidenced by Southern blot analysis) has been reported for human breast carcinomas (102). Additionally, desmocollin appears to be downregulated at both the protein and mRNA level (103). Expression of desmoplakin in breast carcinomas has been variably reported in two separate studies (75, 104) and more research may be required to validate the loss or retention of its expression.

Basal cell carcinomas demonstrate reduced expression of desmoglein and plakoglobin (105). Additionally, plakoglobin expression is also reduced in colon carcinomas (106). More research is needed to examine the expression of other demosomal proteins in human colon carcinomas, including desmoglein, desmocollin and desmoplakin.

2.8.3 Focal Contacts

Focal adhesions (also known as focal contacts) are specialized cell adhesion structures which serve both structural and functional roles in linking the extracellular matrix to the actin cytoskelton during adhesion and migration. Normal tissues demonstrate the presence of focal contacts – an integrin containing multiprotein complex expressed at the cell surface of normal epithelial cells. The components of the focal contact include: the β1 integrin paired with a number of α integrins (including α6, α5 and α3), actin, paxillin, vinculin, talin, laminin-10, nidogen and collagen IV. These structures are thought to be important for cell motility in epithelial cells as has been demonstrated in cell culture systems and wound healing model systems.

Loss of normal β4 integrin expression in prostate carcinoma may lead to increased predominance of α6β1 integrin due to the constitutive synthesis of the α6 and β1 subunits. The α6β1 integrin is a prominent component of the focal adhesion that links the extracellular matrix to the actin cytoskeleton and contributes to transmission of signal transduction and mechanical stability of the cell during matrix remodeling and migration. Unlike the hemidesmosome, the focal adhesion contains more than one integrin subtype. Loss of structural components of the focal adhesion in cell culture studies resulted in defects in membrane blebbing, cell adhesion and spreading and loss of actin stress fibers, highlighting the important role of this adhesion complex in cell motility and adhesion.

An extracellular matrix ligand for α6β1 is the laminin 10/11 isoform, which also functions as a ligand for the α3β1 and α6β4 integrins. Similar to other laminins, the laminin 10/11 isoform is a cruciform complex composed of three subchains: α5, β1 and γ1. Binding of α6β1 integrin by laminin 10/11 facilitates integration of the focal adhesion complex via nidogen into the collagen IV network of the extracellular matrix.

Altered expression of focal adhesion kinase (FAK) has been demonstrated in numerous epithelial tumors. Increased expression of FAK has been reported in prostate via immunohistochemistry (107) and mRNA expression (108) studies and in colon carcinomas by immunohistochemistry (109). Additionally, strong expression of vinculin has been noted in basal cell carcinomas by immunohistochemistry (110) and strong expression of talin in colon carcinomas has also been reported (111).

Conflicting results have been reported in breast carcinomas. Some reports suggest an increase of FAK by immunohistochemistry studies (109) and Western blot analysis (112), while others have reported reduced expression of FAK, including vinculin and talin by immunohistochemistry studies (91). More work is needed in this area to understand the function of the focal adhesion in breast carcinomas.

2.8.4 Other Cell Adhesion Molecules

Tight junctions are simple protein complexes involved in cell adhesion between epithelial cells. They consist of zona occludens 1, and zona occludens 2 proteins. Loss of the tight junction proteins ZO-1 and ZO-2 has been reported in breast carcinomas and pancreatic adenocarcinomas (77, 113).

Microarray analaysis suggested increased expression of CAM in prostate carcinoma (not confirmed by Northern) (41).

3. THE ROLE OF CELL ADHESION IN CANCER METASTASIS

The process of tumor cell metastasis is a multi-step process that has been the subject of great interest in the scientific literature. Not all tumor cells possess the capability to metastasize. In fact it is a rare tumor cell that possesses the ability to successfully metastasize. The process of tumor cell metastasis, while not completely understood, involves the complex modulation of numerous cell processes, including cell adhesion events.

To briefly review, an individual tumor cell must dissociate from the primary tumor mass, presumably due to a combination of altered cell adhesion and proteolytic events. Once free of its cellular attachments, the tumor cell modulates cell adhesion complexes in order to facilitate its movement and invasion through the extracellular stroma. This involves the coordinated release of proteases and expression of extracellular matrix proteins with related cell adhesion molecules to facilitate migration. Eventually, the tumor cell will come into contact with a vascular structure, and gain access to the intra-luminal space by traversing the basement membrane and the endothelial cell junctions of the vessel. According to this view, the tumor cell will travel through the circulation and eventually stop in the capillary bed (or small vessels) of a target organ where it must again pass across the vessel border and extravasate into the extracellular space. The process of a tumor cell leaving a vessel is thought to be very similar to leukocyte extravasation. This involves attachment to an endothelial cell and extension of pseudopodia between the endothelial intercellular junction. The cells retract and the basement membrane is exposed for proteolytic digestion by the tumor cell. Thus, the tumor cell is able to traverse the vascular barrier to begin proliferating in a new environment. As the cell begins to proliferate and multiply, it will begin modifying its environment by changing and/or laying down new extracellular matrix proteins.

4. EXPRESSION OF ADHESION STRUCTURES IN METASTATIC LESIONS

Epithelial tumors frequently metastasize to lymph nodes and other organs. A recent review article of lymph node metastasis postulated three mechanisms which may occur during this process (114). Tumor cells may be trapped in the 'filtering' actions of the lymph node; they may specifically adhere with T-cells within the lymph node; and thirdly, cytokines released from the lymph node may function to alter expression of adhesion molecules in the tumor cell itself. Numerous studies have examined expression of cell adhesion proteins in metastatic lesions. Some examples are discussed below.

Prostate and breast carcinomas frequently metastasize to bone. Two studies have implicated a role for CD44 in facilitating adherence of tumor cells to bone marrow cells in micrometastatic lesions (115,116). Additionally, a mouse model system has helped to elucidate the CD44 interaction with hyaluronan in lung tissue, which facilitates metastasis in a spontaneously metastazising breast carcinoma cell line (117).

While CD44 appears to be important for metastasize in some studies, decreased expression may be important for tumor cell migration and invasion. Invasive micropapillary carcinoma of the breast is an aggressive tumor with a high metastatic potential. Decreased expression of CD44 was identified in 39% of invasive micropapillary carcinomas, compared with only 4% of non-invasive tubular carcinomas and was associated with lymphovascular invasion and lymph node metastasis (118). Modulation of CD44 throughout the tumor cell metastasis process may occur and more studies in this area might help to understand its role.

In breast carcinoma patients, soluble levels of E-selectin, ICAM-1 and VCAM-1 were significantly elevated in the serum of patients with late stage disease, compared with age-matched patients with benign breast disease. Furthermore, elevated expression of VCAM-1 was predictive of decreased survival (119).

In a study of 114 resected colon carcinomas, decreased expression of the $\alpha3$ integrin was positively associated with lymph node metastasis and tumor stage. Furthermore, decreased expression of $\alpha3$ integrin was associated with significantly lower disease-free survival rates for patients, compared with those whose tumors expressed $\alpha3$ integrin. This was also true for patients with lymph node negative tumors (120).

Nanashima and others examined the expression of CD44-v6 and E-cadherin in primary colorectal carcinomas and hepatic metastases. Their data revealed the expression of E-cadherin was significantly lower in the group of primary colorectal carcinomas which metastasized compared with the non-metastasizing carcinomas, and was low in the metastatic liver lesions. Whereas the expression of CD44v6 was significantly higher in the metastatic colorectal primary tumors, compared with non-metastatic tumors and the expression was high in metastatic liver tumors. Loss of expression of E-cadherin was a poor prognostic factor for survival after hepatic resection (121).

Loss of E-cadherin was significantly associated with lymph node metastasis ($p=0.011$) in a study of gastric carcinoma and lymph node micrometastasis (122).

In a cohort study of 200 primary head and neck squamous cell carcinomas and 56 lymph node metastases, expression of E-cadherin was decreased but not entirely lost in primary tumors and the metastatic lesions. However loss of E-cadherin was significantly associated with regional lymph node and distant metastasis and as well as local recurrences, but this association was independent of tumor grade, stage, site, or TNM status. Other desmosomal proteins (desmoplakin, desmoglein) were not shown to be associated with follow up events (123).

Takayama and others examined 71 primary esophageal squamous cell carcinomas and their corresponding lymph node metastases using immunohistochemistry. There was a significant association ($p<0.05$) with decreased cell adhesion molecule (E-cadherin, β-catenin, CD44, CD44-v6, and β1 integrin) expression and the degree of depth of invasion and lymph node metastasis. Furthermore, reduced expression of E-cadherin, β-catenin, and CD44-v6 was found to correlate with increased number of lymph node metastases ($p<0.01$) (124).

5. INHERITED ALTERATIONS IN ADHESION MOLECULES – ASSOCIATED WITH INCREASED RISK FOR CERTAIN CARCINOMAS

There is abundant evidence in the literature that alteration of adhesion structures accompanies and contributes to the progression of epithelial cancers. It is interesting to note that several inherited mutations that ultimately result in the disruption, attenuation or complete loss of the hemidesmosome structure are associated with increased risk of developing certain types of tumors. It is not yet clear whether or not inherited defects in other cell adhesion molecules might also contribute to an increased risk of carcinoma.

5.1 Genetic Blistering Skin Diseases

Epidermolysis bullosa is a rare genetic skin disease that is clinically heterogeneous. Mutations in any of nine different genes (α6 and β4 integrin subunits, α3β3γ2 [332] subunits of laminin-5, BP180, collagen VII, keratin 5 and 14) encoding major protein components of the hemidesmosome (with the exception of BP230) can lead to aberrant adhesion between the basal keratinocytes and the basement membrane in skin. The resulting destabilization and/or complete loss of these structures results in a large clinical spectrum of skin fragility, blistering, chronic wound healing, deformation and even death. Studies in the literature and case reports suggest these patients are cancer prone, and are at increased risk of developing squamous cell carcinomas of the skin. Interestingly, not all skin cancers are increased in incidence. The incidence of basal cell carcinoma in this patient population, is actually lower than in the general population (125), yet there is a slightly increased risk of developing melanoma in these patient populations (126).

Analysis of the National Epidermolysis Bullosa Registry (NEBR) has been unable to make a significant correlation with development of extracutaneous malignancies in these patients. This may be due to premature death in the patient population (126). Several case reports do exist however, including osteogenic sarcoma of the tibia (127), squamous cell carcinoma of the hard palate (128), esophageal squamous cell carcinoma (129), breast carcinoma (130) and cervical cancer (131).

The diseases are defined biologically, based on the ultrastructural level of separation that occurs in the skin; intraepidermal, lamina lucida, or sub-lamina densa. As with most disease types, recent publications suggest there is a large degree of overlap among the phenotypical presentation and ultimately the biological abnormality.

5.2 EB VARIANTS

5.2.1 Dystrophic

Dystrophic epidermolysis bullosa (DEB) is a particularly destructive subset of the EB disease types that results in blistering, scarring and severe deformation. This variant can be inherited either autosomal dominantly or autosomal recessively. Mutations occur in the gene encoding collagen VII and ultrastructural tissue separation occurs at the sub-lamina densa. There are at least 192 different mutations described in the collagen VII gene which result in clinically apparent disease. Mutations in collagen VII gene were first described in 1993 (132, 133). Examination of the human gene mutation database reveals most of these mutations are missense/nonsense nucleotide substitutions. Cumulative data suggests a "hotspot" mutation exists in COL7A1, G2043R (134). These patients are at 76% increased cumulative risk for developing and dying from SCC (135). Although usually histologically well-differentiated, most of the SCCs in these patients are clinically highly aggressive. Local recurrence is common, as is regional spread and eventual metastasis and death (126).

It is interesting to note that many patients with blistering disease subtypes will improve as they age. This suggests the body may be capable of developing a tolerance and/or compensatory mechanisms to compensate for genetic mutation in some hemidesmosome components. With the genetic loss of collagen VII, the hemidesmosome is without an anchoring fibril and compensation of such an integral part of the hemidesmosome would seem less likely. This may in part, explain the extremely high incidence of SCC in DEB patients.

5.2.2 Junctional

Junctional epidermolysis bullosa (JEB) involves blistering that is ultrastructurally apparent in the lamina lucida of the basement membrane zone. The clinical severity is often lethal in this subtype of disease, Herlitz JEB. Mutations in all three laminin-5 subunits (α3, β3 and γ2) have been described. Mutations in the α3 subunit of laminin-5 were first reported in 1995 (136, 137). Now there are four mutations which have been described in total, three of which are small deletions. Mutations in the β3 subunit of laminin-5 were first reported in 1994 (138), since then there are at least 41 different mutations which have been reported. The majority of the mutations that have been reported are found in the β3 subunit (LAMB3) (139). Two 'hotspot' mutations have emerged in the literature, R635X and R42X (140, 141) which account for nearly half of the described mutations in patient samples in one study (13/20 patient samples examined). Mutations in the γ2 subunit of laminin-5 were first reported in 1994 (142-144). Now there are at least 14 described mutations that result in clinically apparent disease.

Genetic mutations in several other hemidesmosome proteins have also been described and are considered as three distinct subtypes of JEB. Clinical severity is highly variable depending on the nature of the mutation. In these patients, the ultrastructural defect that accompanies blistering occurs at the basal keratinocyte/lamina lucida interface.

Generalized atrophic benign epidermolysis bullosa (also known as JEB non-Herlitz subtype) occurs due to mutations in the gene encoding BP180 (collagen XVII). At least 27 different mutations have been described, the first report occurring in 1995 (145), the majority of which are nucleotide substitutions and small deletions. Mutations in either the α6 or β4 integrin subunits lead to a neonatal lethal variant of EB termed epidermolysis bullosa with pyloric atresia. Three mutations have been reported in the α6 integrin, the first of which was reported in 1997 (146, 147). In contrast, at least 32 different mutations have been described in the β4 integrin subunit which result in clinically apparent disease. Mutations the in β4 integrin subunit were first reported in 1995 (148) and there are at least 32 different mutations which have been reported. One study demonstrated that two different mutations in the β4 integrin tail could result in a loss of the ability to recruit plectin in hemidesmosome formation (149). Epidermolysis bullosa associated with late onset muscular dystrophy has been reported to be the result of a mutation in the cytoplasmic protein plectin. Mutations in this gene were first reported in 1996 (150-153) and there are at least 22 different mutations reported in the literature.

Many of these mutations result in early embryonic lethal clinical outcomes, yet there are several case reports that suggest there is an increased risk of development of squamous cell carcinoma in this patient population as well (154-157). Too few case reports have been made to calculate accurate lifetime risk of developing squamous cell carcinoma (126). One possible explanation for why more squamous cell carcinomas are not seen is the high degree of lethality at a young age with this disease. The percentage of death in JEB patients collectively from age 1-25 is consistently higher than even the most lethal form of epidermolysis bullosa (dystrophic) in this age group (126), which may partially explain the discrepancy in development of SCC in JEB patients.

5.2.3 Simplex

Epidermolysis bullosa simplex (EB) involves blistering due to fragility of the basal cell layer of the keratinocytes. Upon ultrastructural examination, the level of tissue separation is found to occur intraepidermally, within the basal keratinocyte itself, generally within the subnuclear cytoplasm. There are three different clinical variants which are described and vary by clinical severity: EBS-Weber Cockayne, EBS-Kobner and EBS- Dowling Meara. Mutations in either keratin 5 or keratin 14 may lead to this disease subtype. The first report of a genetic mutation in the KRT5 gene came in 1992 (158), and now there are at least 25 different mutations that have been described. A genetic mutation in KRT14, the gene encoding the keratin 14 protein, was first described in 1991 (159, 160). Now there are at least 26 different mutations that have been described that result in clinically apparent disease. With increased scrutiny of this patient population, 'hotspot' mutations have now become apparent. A report by Ehrlich and others in 1995 found an Ile to Ser substitution in codon 161 in keratin 5 in six out of thirteen cases examined (161). Studies on keratin 14 have also revealed a 'hotspot' mutation at Arg 125 which occurs in the highly conserved helix initiation peptide (160, 162-164). A mutation in the conserved helix termination peptide was also described for keratin 5 (158). The majority of mutations described (missense/nonsense) appear to cluster in the conserved helix boundary motifs of keratin. By age 60, these patients are only at a slightly increased risk (1.4%) for developing cutaneous squamous cell carcinomas compared with the general population (130).

5.2.4 Xeroderma Pigmentosum

Another example of genetic disease, which leaves the patient at increased risk of cancer, is the condition known as xeroderma pigmentosum (XP), which results from a defect in nucleotide excision repair. These patients have severe deficiency in the nucleotide excision repair of UV radiation induced DNA lesions. This results in changes in pigmentation and an increased frequency of skin cancers. Bernerd et al. (165) reported an increased deposition of α6 and β1 integrins in the basement membrane zone of the skin in XP patients. The skin was more proliferative and invasive. As the α6 integrin binds to either β1 or β4 subunits, this study suggests that the balance between α6β1 and α6β4 integrins are perturbed in these patients, although more studies will need to be done to confirm this question. These findings suggest that alteration of the basement membrane integrins may accompany and even predispose patients to developing cancer. Furthermore, XP keratinocytes grow more quickly and more rapidly than non-XP controls (166).

6. FUTURE STRATEGIES FOR CANCER THERAPY SURROGATE ENDPOINT BIOMARKERS

We have demonstrated that in prostate tumors, the adhesion proteins that are part of the hemidesmosome are early changes. They are first recognizable as early as the precancerous Prostatic Intraepithelial Neoplasia (PIN) lesions – thus appearing before many of the reported genomic perturbations in prostate cancer such as p53 and Rb protein mutations.

Research in prostate cancer, as well as numerous other epithelial cancers, would benefit greatly from increased knowledge of the genetic blistering skin diseases such as mutation analysis. While many different mutations have been described, it would be important to understand which, if any, recurring mutations could be correlated with increased risk of tumors in patients. This information could then be systematically applied to other research areas in epithelial tumor progression. Additionally, correlation of any 'hotspot' mutations with epithelial tumor progression would be important. Identification of any 'hotspot' mutations would be potentially important in identifying one cause of epithelial tumor progression.

Accumulation of genetic mutations in these important protein complexes may result in a tendency towards tumor progression. This may be one mechanism for loss of protein function in these tumors. Other mechanisms may also be important such as gene silencing of key protein components.

It would be potentially interesting to determine which of the described mutations in the genetic skin diseases are most closely associated with patients developing skin tumors. This data could be correlated into identifying possible 'hotspot' mutations of the hemidesmosome proteins.

With new technologies such as microarray, much new data is being brought to light each day in tumor biology research. Automated mutation analysis for the inherited mutations found in blistering skin diseases may one day contribute towards searching for mutations in epithelial tumors. As pharmacogenomics is increasingly becoming a topic of interest, perhaps the combination of these with hemidesmosome tumor mutation screening may one day contribute to better diagnosis and treatment options for patients.

REFERENCES

1. Van den Bergh, F., Giudice, G.J. BP180 (type XVII collagen) and its role in cutaneousbiology and disease. Adv Dermatol, 2003; 19:37-71.
2. Sterk, L.M., Geuijen, C.A., Van den Bergh, J.G., Claessen, N., Weening, J.J., Sonnenberg, A. Association of the tetraspanin CD151 with the laminin-binding integrins alpha3beta1,alpha6beta1, alpha6beta4 and alph7beta1 in cells in culture and in vivo. J Cell Sci2002.June 15:115(pt12):2615.
3. Koster, J., van Wilpe, S., Kuikman, I., Litjens, S.H., Sonnenberg, A. Role of binding ofplectin to the integrin beta4 subunit in the assembly of hemidesmosomes. Mol Biol Cell,2004 Mar; 15(3):1211-23. Epub 2003 Dec.
4. Hynes, R.O. Integrins: bidirectional, allosteric signaling machines. Cell. 2002 Sep 20;110(6):673-87.
5. Nievers, M.G., Kuikman I., Geerts, D., Leigh, I.M., Sonnenberg, A. Formation of hemidesmosome-like structures in the absence of ligand binding by the (alph) 6(beta)4integrin requires binding of HD1/plectin to the cytoplasmic domain of the (beta)4 integrinsubunit. J Cell Sci. 2000 Mar; 113 (Pt 6):963-73.
6. Nagle, R.B., et al., Expression of hemidesmosomal and extracellular matrix proteins bynormal and malignant human prostate tissue. Am J Pathol, 1995. 146(6): p. 1498-507.
7. Cress, A.E., et al., The alpha 6 beta 1 and alpha 6 beta 4 integrins in human prostate cancer progression. Cancer Metastasis Rev, 1995. 14(3): p. 219-28.
8. Knox, J.D., et al., Differential expression of extracellular matrix molecules and the alpha 6-integrins in the normal and neoplastic prostate. Am J Pathol, 1994. 145(1): p. 167-74.
9. Nagle, R.B., et al., Adhesion molecules, extracellular matrix, and proteases in prostate carcinoma. J Cell Biochem Suppl, 1994. 19: p. 232-7.
10. Bonkhoff, H., Analytical molecular pathology of epithelial-stromal interactions in the normal and neoplastic prostate. Anal Quant Cytol Histol, 1998. 20(5): p. 437-42.

11. Allen, M.V., et al., Downregulation of the beta4 integrin subunit in prostatic carcinoma and prostatic intraepithelial neoplasia. Hum Pathol, 1998. 29(4): p. 311-8.
12. Bonkhoff, H., Stein, U. and Remberger, K. Differential expression of alpha 6 and alpha 2 very late antigen integrins in the normal, hyperplastic, and neoplastic prostate: simultaneous demonstration of cell surface receptors and their extracellular ligands. Hum Pathol, 1993. 24(3): p. 243-8.
13. Davis, T.L., et al., Unique expression pattern of the alpha6beta4 integrin and laminin-5 in human prostate carcinoma. Prostate, 2001. 46(3): p. 240-8.
14. Tagliabue, E., et al., Prognostic value of alpha 6 beta 4 integrin expression in breast carcinomas is affected by laminin production from tumor cells. Clin Cancer Res, 1998. 4(2): p. 407-10.
15. Jones, J.L., Critchley, D.R. and Walker, R.A. Alteration of stromal protein and integrin expression in breast--a marker of premalignant change? J Pathol, 1992. 167(4): p. 399-406.
16. Bahadoran, P., et al., Altered expression of the hemidesmosome-anchoring filament complex proteins in basal cell carcinoma: possible role in the origin of peritumoral lacunae. Br J Dermatol, 1997. 136(1): p. 35-42.
17. Chopra, A., Maitra, B. and Korman, N.J. Decreased mRNA expression of several basement membrane components in basal cell carcinoma. J Invest Dermatol, 1998. 110(1): p. 52-6.
18. Dumas, V., et al., Expression of basement membrane antigens and matrix metalloproteinases 2 and 9 in cutaneous basal and squamous cell carcinomas. Anticancer Res, 1999. 19(4B): p. 2929-38.
19. Herold-Mende, C., et al., Metastatic growth of squamous cell carcinomas is correlated with upregulation and redistribution of hemidesmosomal components. Cell Tissue Res, 2001. 306(3): p. 399-408.
20. Tennenbaum, T., et al., Extracellular matrix receptors and mouse skin carcinogenesis: altered expression linked to appearance of early markers of tumor progression. Cancer Res, 1992. 52(10): p. 2966-76.
21. Witkowski, C.M., et al., Altered surface expression and increased turnover of the alpha6beta4 integrin in an undifferentiated carcinoma. Carcinogenesis, 2000. 21(2): p. 325-30.
22. Garzino-Demo, P., et al., Altered expression of alpha 6 integrin subunit in oral squamous cell carcinoma and oral potentially malignant lesions. Oral Oncol, 1998. 34(3): p. 204-10.
23. Skubitz, A.P., et al., Expression of alpha 6 and beta 4 integrins in serous ovarian carcinoma correlates with expression of the basement membrane protein laminin. Am J Pathol, 1996. 148(5): p. 1445-61.
24. Carlevato, M.T., et al., Differential integrin expression in thyroid and laryngeal carcinomas. Anticancer Res, 1996. 16(4C): p. 2379-84.
25. Pouliot, N., Nice, E.C., and Burgess, A.W. Laminin-10 mediates basal and EGF-stimulated motility of human colon carcinoma cells via alpha(3)beta(1) and alpha(6)beta(4) integrins. Exp Cell Res, 2001. 266(1): p. 1-10.
26. Lohi, J., et al., Basement membrane laminin-5 is deposited in colorectal adenomas and carcinomas and serves as a ligand for alpha3beta1 integrin. Apmis, 2000. 108(3): p. 161-72.
27. Fontao, L., et al., Polarized expression of HD1: relationship with the cytoskeleton in cultured human colonic carcinoma cells. Exp Cell Res, 1997. 231(2): p. 319-27.
28. Chao, C., et al., A function for the integrin alpha6beta4 in the invasive properties of colorectal carcinoma cells. Cancer Res, 1996. 56(20): p. 4811-9.

29. Van Waes, C., et al., The A9 antigen associated with aggressive human squamous carcinoma is structurally and functionally similar to the newly defined integrin alpha 6 beta 4. Cancer Res, 1991. 51(9): p. 2395-402.
30. Sordat, I., et al., Differential expression of laminin-5 subunits and integrin receptors in human colorectal neoplasia. J Pathol, 1998. 185(1): p. 44-52.
31. Stallmach, A., et al., Diminished expression of integrin adhesion molecules on human colonic epithelial cells during the benign to malign tumour transformation. Gut, 1992. 33(3): p. 342-6.
32. Geuijen, C.A. and Sonnenberg, A. Dynamics of the alpha6beta4 Integrin in Keratinocytes. Mol Biol Cell, 2002. 13(11): p. 3845-58.
33. Tsuruta, D., Hopkinson, S.B., and Jones, J.C. Hemidesmosome protein dynamics in live epithelial cells. Cell Motil Cytoskeleton, 2003. 54(2): p. 122-34.
34. Uematsu, J., et al., Demonstration of type II hemidesmosomes in a mammary gland epithelial cell line, BMGE-H. J Biochem (Tokyo), 1994. 115(3): p. 469-76.
35. Fontao, L., et al., Regulation of the type II hemidesmosomal plaque assembly in intestinal epithelial cells. Exp Cell Res, 1999. 250(2): p. 298-312.
36. Hieda, Y., et al., Identification of a new hemidesmosomal protein, HD1: a major, high molecular mass component of isolated hemidesmosomes. J Cell Biol, 1992. 116(6): p. 1497-506.
37. Posteraro, P., DeLuca, N., Meneguzzi, G., El Hachem, M., Angelo, C., Gobello, T., Tadini, G., Zambruno, G., Castiglia, D. Laminin-5 mutational analysis in an Italian cohort of patients with junctional epidermolysis bullosa. J Invest Dermatol, 2004 Oct;123(4):xii-xiii.
38. Rousselle, P., et al., Laminin 5 binds the NC-1 domain of type VII collagen. J Cell Biol, 1997. 138(3): p. 719-28.
39. Hao, J., et al., Differential expression of laminin 5 (alpha 3 beta 3 gamma 2) by human malignant and normal prostate. Am J Pathol, 1996. 149(4): p. 1341-9.
40. Hao, J., et al., Investigation into the mechanism of the loss of laminin 5 (alpha3beta3-gamma2) expression in prostate cancer. Am J Pathol, 2001. 158(3): p. 1129-35.
41. Ernst, T., et al., Decrease and gain of gene expression are equally discriminatory markers for prostate carcinoma: a gene expression analysis on total and microdissected prostate tissue. Am J Pathol, 2002. 160(6): p. 2169-80.
42. Maatta, M., et al., Comparative analysis of the distribution of laminin chains in the basement membranes in some malignant epithelial tumors: the alpha1 chain of laminin shows a selected expression pattern in human carcinomas. J Histochem Cytochem, 2001. 49(6): p. 711-26.
43. Daigo, Y., et al., Degenerate oligonucleotide primed-polymerase chain reaction-based array comparative genomic hybridization for extensive amplicon profiling of breast cancers : a new approach for the molecular analysis of paraffin-embedded cancer tissue. Am J Pathol, 2001. 158(5): p. 1623-31.
44. Aoki, S., et al., Prognostic significance of laminin-5 gamma2 chain expression in colorectal carcinoma: immunohistochemical analysis of 103 cases. Dis Colon Rectum, 2002. 45(11): p. 1520-7.
45. Li, K., et al., Cloning of partial cDNA for mouse 180-kDa bullous pemphigoid antigen (BPAG2), a highly conserved collagenous protein of the cutaneous basement membrane zone. J Invest Dermatol, 1992. 99(3): p. 258-63.
46. Hopkinson, S.B. and Jones, J.C. The N terminus of the transmembrane protein BP180 interacts with the N-terminal domain of BP230, thereby mediating keratin cytoskeleton

anchorage to the cell surface at the site of the hemidesmosome. Mol Biol Cell, 2000. 11(1): p. 277-86.
47. Koster, J., et al., Analysis of the interactions between BP180, BP230, plectin and the integrin alpha6beta4 important for hemidesmosome assembly. J Cell Sci, 2003. 116(Pt 2): p. 387-399.
48. Hopkinson, S.B., Baker, S.E., and Jones, J.C. Molecular genetic studies of a human epidermal autoantigen (the 180-kD bullous pemphigoid antigen/BP180): identification of functionally important sequences within the BP180 molecule and evidence for an interaction between BP180 and alpha 6 integrin. J Cell Biol, 1995. 130(1): p. 117-25.
49. Hopkinson, S.B., et al., Interaction of BP180 (type XVII collagen) and alpha6 integrin is necessary for stabilization of hemidesmosome structure. J Invest Dermatol, 1998. 111(6): p. 1015-22.
50. Tanaka, M., et al., Characterization of bullous pemphigoid antibodies by use of recombi-nant bullous pemphigoid antigen proteins. J Invest Dermatol, 1991. 97(4): p. 725-8.
51. Ruhrberg, C. and Watt, F.M. The plakin family: versatile organizers of cytoskeletal architecture. Curr Opin Genet Dev, 1997. 7(3): p. 392-7.
52. Bergstraesser, L.M., et al., Expression of hemidesmosomes and component proteins is lost by invasive breast cancer cells. Am J Pathol, 1995. 147(6): p. 1823-39.
53. Zhu, X.J., Niimi, Y., and Bystryn, J.C. Identification of a 160-kD molecule as a component of the basement membrane zone and as a minor bullous pemphigoid antigen. J Invest Dermatol, 1990. 94(6): p. 817-21.
54. Fairley, J.A., et al., Expression pattern of the bullous pemphigoid-180 antigen in normal and neoplastic epithelia. Br J Dermatol, 1995. 133(3): p. 385-91.
55. Yamada, T., et al., Aberrant expression of a hemidesmosomal protein, bullous pemphigoid antigen 2, in human squamous cell carcinoma. Lab Invest, 1996. 75(4): p. 589-600.
56. Schaapveld, R.Q., et al., Hemidesmosome formation is initiated by the beta4 integrin subunit, requires complex formation of beta4 and HD1/plectin, and involves a direct interaction between beta4 and the bullous pemphigoid antigen 180. J Cell Biol, 1998. 142(1): p. 271-84.
57. Burgeson, R.E., Type VII collagen, anchoring fibrils, and epidermolysis bullosa. J Invest Dermatol, 1993. 101(3): p. 252-5.
58. Keene, D.R., et al., Type VII collagen forms an extended network of anchoring fibrils. J Cell Biol, 1987. 104(3): p. 611-21.
59. Liebert, M., et al., Loss of co-localization of alpha 6 beta 4 integrin and collagen VII in bladder cancer. Am J Pathol, 1994. 144(4): p. 787-95.
60. Fuchs, E., Keratins and the skin. Annu Rev Cell Dev Biol, 1995. 11: p. 123-53.
61. Irvine, A.D. and McLean, W.H. Human keratin diseases: the increasing spectrum of disease and subtlety of the phenotype-genotype correlation. Br J Dermatol, 1999. 140(5): p. 815-28.
62. Quinlan, R., Hutchison, C., and Lane, B. Intermediate filament proteins. Protein Profile, 1994. 1(8): p. 779-911.
63. Goldstein, N.S., Immunophenotypic characterization of 225 prostate adenocarcinomas with intermediate or high Gleason scores. Am J Clin Pathol, 2002. 117(3): p. 471-7.
64. Yang, Y., et al., Differential expression of cytokeratin mRNA and protein in normal prostate, prostatic intraepithelial neoplasia, and invasive carcinoma. Am J Pathol, 1997. 150(2): p. 693-704.

65. Abrahams, N.A., Ormsby, A.H. and Brainard, J. Validation of cytokeratin 5/6 as aneffective substitute for keratin 903 in the differentiation of benign from malignant glands in prostate needle biopsies. Histopathology, 2002. 41(1): p. 35-41.
66. Sherwood, E.R., et al., Differential expression of specific cytokeratin polypeptides in the basal and luminal epithelia of the human prostate. Prostate, 1991. 18(4): p. 303-14.
67. Wang, W., et al., Single cell behavior in metastatic primary mammary tumors correlatedwith gene expression patterns revealed by molecular profiling. Cancer Res, 2002. 62(21):p. 6278-88.
68. Tsubura, A., et al., Keratin expression in the normal breast and in breast carcinoma. Histopathology, 1991. 18(6): p. 517-22.
69. Tot, T., The cytokeratin profile of medullary carcinoma of the breast. Histopathology, 2000. 37(2): p. 175-81.
70. Schirren, C.G., et al., Trichoblastoma and basal cell carcinoma are neoplasms with follicular differentiation sharing the same profile of cytokeratin intermediate filaments. Am J Dermatopathol, 1997. 19(4): p. 341-50.
71. Shinohara, M., et al., Immunohistochemical study of desmosomes in oral squamous cellcarcinoma: correlation with cytokeratin and E-cadherin staining, and with tumour behaviour. J Pathol, 1998. 184(4): p. 369-81.
72. Pittella, F., et al., Perinuclear and cytoplasmic distribution of desmoglein in esophageal squamous cell carcinomas. Pathol Res Pract, 2001. 197(2): p. 85-91.
73. Kallakury, B.V., et al., Decreased expression of catenins (alpha and beta), p120 CTN, and E-cadherin cell adhesion proteins and E-cadherin gene promoter methylation in prostatic adenocarcinomas. Cancer, 2001. 92(11): p. 2786-95.
74. Chesire, D.R., et al., Detection and analysis of beta-catenin mutations in prostate cancer. Prostate, 2000. 45(4): p. 323-34.
75. Davies, E.L., et al., The immunohistochemical expression of desmoplakin and its role in vivo in the progression and metastasis of breast cancer. Eur J Cancer, 1999. 35(6): p. 902-7.
76. Sommers, C.L., et al., Alterations in beta-catenin phosphorylation and plakoglobin expression in human breast cancer cells. Cancer Res, 1994. 54(13): p. 3544-52.
77. Hoover, K.B., Liao, S.Y., and Bryant, P.J. Loss of the tight junction MAGUK ZO-1 in breast cancer: relationship to glandular differentiation and loss of heterozygosity. Am J Pathol, 1998. 153(6): p. 1767-73.
78. Yoshiura, K., et al., Silencing of the E-cadherin invasion-suppressor gene by CpG methylation in human carcinomas. Proc Natl Acad Sci U S A, 1995. 92(16): p. 7416-9.
79. Tamura, G., et al., E-Cadherin gene promoter hypermethylation in primary human gastriccarcinomas. J Natl Cancer Inst, 2000. 92(7): p. 569-73.
80. Corn, P.G., et al., Frequent hypermethylation of the 5' CpG island of E-cadherin in esophageal adenocarcinoma. Clin Cancer Res, 2001. 7(9): p. 2765-9.
81. Azarschab, P., et al., Epigenetic control of E-cadherin (CDH1) by CpG methylation in metastasising laryngeal cancer. Oncol Rep, 2003. 10(2): p. 501-3.
82. Droufakou, S., et al., Multiple ways of silencing E-cadherin gene expression in lobular carcinoma of the breast. Int J Cancer, 2001. 92(3): p. 404-8.
83. Hazan, R.B., et al., Cadherin switch in tumor progression. Ann N Y Acad Sci, 2004. 1014: p. 155-63.
84. Rubin, M.A., et al., E-cadherin expression in prostate cancer: a broad survey using high-density tissue microarray technology. Hum Pathol, 2001. 32(7): p. 690-7.

85. Aho, S., et al., Specific sequences in p120ctn determine subcellular distribution of its multiple isoforms involved in cellular adhesion of normal and malignant epithelial cells. J Cell Sci, 2002. 115(Pt 7): p. 1391-402.
86. Kallakury, B.V., Sheehan, C.E. and Ross, J.S. Co-downregulation of cell adhesion proteins alpha- and beta-catenins, p120CTN, E-cadherin, and CD44 in prostatic adenocarcinomas. Hum Pathol, 2001. 32(8): p. 849-55.
87. Arenas, M.I., et al., E-, N- and P-cadherin, and alpha-, beta- and gamma-catenin protein expression in normal, hyperplastic and carcinomatous human prostate. Histochem J, 2000. 32(11): p. 659-67.
88. Moll, R., et al., Differential loss of E-cadherin expression in infiltrating ductal and lobular breast carcinomas. Am J Pathol, 1993. 143(6): p. 1731-42.
89. Rimm, D.L., Sinard, J.H., and Morrow, J.S. Reduced alpha-catenin and E-cadherin expression in breast cancer. Lab Invest, 1995. 72(5): p. 506-12.
90. Dillon, D.A., et al., The expression of p120ctn protein in breast cancer is independent of alpha- and beta-catenin and E-cadherin. Am J Pathol, 1998. 152(1): p. 75-82.
91. Glukhova, M., et al., Adhesion systems in normal breast and in invasive breast carcinoma. Am J Pathol, 1995. 146(3): p. 706-16.
92. Pizarro, A., E-cadherin expression is frequently reduced in infiltrative basal cell carcinoma. J Dermatol, 2000. 27(12): p. 804-5.
93. Kooy, A.J., et al., Expression of E-cadherin, alpha- & beta-catenin, and CD44V6 and the subcellular localization of E-cadherin and CD44V6 in normal epidermis and basal cell carcinoma. Hum Pathol, 1999. 30(11): p. 1328-35.
94. Yamazaki, F., et al., Immunohistochemical detection for nuclear beta-catenin in sporadic basal cell carcinoma. Br J Dermatol, 2001. 145(5): p. 771-7.
95. Boonchai, W., et al., Expression of beta-catenin, a key mediator of the WNT signaling pathway, in basal cell carcinoma. Arch Dermatol, 2000. 136(7): p. 937-8.
96. Schuhmacher, C., et al., Loss of immunohistochemical E-cadherin expression in colon cancer is not due to structural gene alterations. Virchows Arch, 1999. 434(6): p. 489-95.
97. Hiscox, S. and Jiang, W.G. Expression of E-cadherin, alpha, beta and gamma-catenin in human colorectal cancer. Anticancer Res, 1997. 17(2B): p. 1349-54.
98. Raftopoulos, I., et al., Level of alpha-catenin expression in colorectal cancer correlates with invasiveness, metastatic potential, and survival. J Surg Oncol, 1998. 68(2): p. 92-9.
99. Sellin, J.H., et al., Increased beta-catenin expression and nuclear translocation accompany cellular hyperproliferation in vivo. Cancer Res, 2001. 61(7): p. 2899-906.
100. Takemasa, I., et al., Construction of preferential cDNA microarray specialized for human colorectal carcinoma: molecular sketch of colorectal cancer. Biochem Biophys Res Commun, 2001. 285(5): p. 1244-9.
101. Schmelz, M., et al., PEAZ-1: a new human prostate neoplastic epithelial cell line. Prostate, 2001. 48(2): p. 79-92.
102. Aberle, H., et al., The human plakoglobin gene localizes on chromosome 17q21 and is subjected to loss of heterozygosity in breast and ovarian cancers. Proc Natl Acad Sci U S A, 1995. 92(14): p. 6384-8.
103. Klus, G.T., et al., Down-regulation of the desmosomal cadherin desmocollin 3 in human breast cancer. Int J Oncol, 2001. 19(1): p. 169-74.
104. Dervan, P.A., et al., Desmosomal plaque proteins are preserved in all grades of breast cancer. An immunohistochemical study utilizing monoclonal antibodies to desmoplakin. Am J Surg Pathol, 1988. 12(11): p. 855-60.
105. Tada, H., et al., Expression of desmoglein I and plakoglobin in skin carcinomas. J Cutan Pathol, 2000. 27(1): p. 24-9.

106. Lifschitz-Mercer, B., et al., Nuclear Localization of beta-Catenin and Plakoglobin in Primary and Metastatic Human Colonic Carcinomas, Colonic Adenomas, and Normal Colon. Int J Surg Pathol, 2001. 9(4): p. 273-9.
107. Rovin, J.D., et al., Expression of focal adhesion kinase in normal and pathologic human prostate tissues. Prostate, 2002. 53(2): p. 124-32.
108. Weiner, T.M., et al., Expression of focal adhesion kinase gene and invasive cancer. Lancet, 1993. 342(8878): p. 1024-5.
109. Cance, W.G., et al., Immunohistochemical analyses of focal adhesion kinase expression in benign and malignant human breast and colon tissues: correlation with preinvasive and invasive phenotypes. Clin Cancer Res, 2000. 6(6): p. 2417-23.
110. Lifschitz-Mercer, B., et al., Expression of the adherens junction protein vinculin in human basal and squamous cell tumors: relationship to invasiveness and metastatic potential. Hum Pathol, 1997. 28(11): p. 1230-6.
111. Porter, R.M., et al., Monoclonal antibodies to cytoskeletal proteins: an immunohistochemical investigation of human colon cancer. J Pathol, 1993. 170(4): p. 435-40.
112. Owens, L.V., et al., Overexpression of the focal adhesion kinase (p125FAK) in invasive human tumors. Cancer Res, 1995. 55(13): p. 2752-5.
113. Chlenski, A., et al., Organization and expression of the human zo-2 gene (tjp-2) in normal and neoplastic tissues. Biochem Biophys Acta, 2000. 1493(3): p. 319-24.
114. Gendreau, K.M. and Whalen, G.F. What can we learn from the phenomenon of preferential lymph node metastasis in carcinoma? J Surg Oncol, 1999. 70(3): p. 199-204.
115. Draffin, J.E., et al., CD44 potentiates the adherence of metastatic prostate and breast cancer cells to bone marrow endothelial cells. Cancer Res, 2004. 64(16): p. 5702-11.
116. Hill, A., et al., The emerging role of CD44 in regulating skeletal micrometastasis. Cancer Lett, 2005.
117. Lopez, J.I., et al., CD44 attenuates metastatic invasion during breast cancer progression. Cancer Res, 2005. 65(15): p. 6755-63.
118. Gong, Y., et al., Expression of cell adhesion molecules, CD44s and E-cadherin, and microvessel density in invasive micropapillary carcinoma of the breast. Histopathology, 2005. 46(1): p. 24-30.
119. O'Hanlon, D.M., et al., Soluble adhesion molecules (E-selectin, ICAM-1 and VCAM-1) in breast carcinoma. Eur J Cancer, 2002. 38(17): p. 2252-7.
120. Hashida, H., et al., Integrin alpha3 expression as a prognostic factor in colon cancer: association with MRP-1/CD9 and KAI1/CD82. Int J Cancer, 2002. 97(4): p. 518-25.
121. Nanashima, A., et al., Expression of adhesion molecules in hepatic metastases of colorectal carcinoma: relationship to primary tumours and prognosis after hepatic resection. J Gastroenterol Hepatol, 1999. 14(10): p. 1004-9.
122. Wu, Z.Y., et al., Expression of E-cadherin in gastric carcinoma and its correlation with lymph node micrometastasis. World J Gastroenterol, 2005. 11(20): p. 3139-43.
123. Bosch, F.X., et al., E-cadherin is a selective and strongly dominant prognostic factor in squamous cell carcinoma: a comparison of E-cadherin with desmosomal components. Int J Cancer, 2005. 114(5): p. 779-90.
124. Takayama, N., et al., Relationship between the expression of adhesion molecules in primary esophageal squamous cell carcinoma and metastatic lymph nodes. Anticancer Res, 2003. 23(6a): p. 4435-42.
125. Lear, J.T. and Smith, A.G. Basal cell carcinoma. Postgrad Med J, 1997. 73(863): p. 538- 42.

126. Fine, J., et al., Epidermolysis bullosa: clinical, epidemiologic, and laboratory advances and the findings of the national epidermolysis bullosa registry. 1999, Baltimore: Johns Hopkins University Press.
127. Yamauchi, Y., Takahashi, K. and Shiotsu, H. Osteogenic sarcoma of the tibia in a patient with epidermolysis bullosa dystrophica. Clin Orthop, 1988(228): p. 273-7.
128. Martinez, L., Goodman, P. and Crow, W.N. Squamous cell carcinoma of the maxillary sinus and palate in epidermolysis bullosa: CT demonstration. J Comput Assist Tomogr, 1992. 16(2): p. 317-9.
129. Horn, H.M. and Tidman, M.J. The clinical spectrum of dystrophic epidermolysis bullosa. Br J Dermatol, 2002. 146(2): p. 267-74.
130. Lyons, J.A., et al., Successful Breast Conservation in a Patient with Epidermolysis Bullosa Simplex. Breast J, 1999. 5(6): p. 404-406.
131. Etienne, A., et al., [Epidermolysis bullosa acquisita and metastatic cancer of the uterine cervix]. Ann Dermatol Venereol, 1998. 125(5): p. 321-3.
132. Christiano, A.M., et al., Mutation-based prenatal diagnosis of Herlitz junctional pidermolysis bullosa. Prenat Diagn, 1997. 17(4): p. 343-54.
133. Hilal, L., et al., A homozygous insertion-deletion in the type VII collagen gene (COL7A1) in Hallopeau-Siemens dystrophic epidermolysis bullosa. Nat Genet, 1993. 5(3): p. 287-93.
134. Mellerio, J.E., et al., A recurrent glycine substitution mutation, G2043R, in the type VII collagen gene (COL7A1) in dominant dystrophic epidermolysis bullosa. Br J Dermatol, 1998. 139(4): p. 730-7.
135. Mallipeddi, R., Epidermolysis bullosa and cancer. Clin Exp Dermatol, 2002. 27(8): p. 616-23.
136. McGrath, J.A., et al., A homozygous nonsense mutation in the alpha 3 chain gene of laminin 5 (LAMA3) in Herlitz junctional epidermolysis bullosa: prenatal exclusion in a fetus at risk. Genomics, 1995. 29(1): p. 282-4.
137. Vidal, F., et al., Cloning of the laminin alpha 3 chain gene (LAMA3) and identification of a homozygous deletion in a patient with Herlitz junctional epidermolysis bullosa. Genomics, 1995. 30(2): p. 273-80.
138. Plkkinen, L., et al., Cloning of the beta 3 chain gene (LAMB3) of human laminin 5, a candidate gene in junctional epidermolysis bullosa. Genomics, 1995. 25(1): p. 192-8.139.
139. Pulkkinen, L. and J. Uitto, Mutation analysis and molecular genetics of epidermolysis bullosa. Matrix Biol, 1999. 18(1): p. 29-42.
140. Kivirikko, S., et al., Mutational hotspots in the LAMB3 gene in the lethal (Herlitz) type of junctional epidermolysis bullosa. Hum Mol Genet, 1996. 5(2): p. 231-7.
141. Pulkkinen, L., et al., Predominance of the recurrent mutation R635X in the LAMB3 gene in European patients with Herlitz junctional epidermolysis bullosa has implications for mutation detection strategy. J Invest Dermatol, 1997. 109(2): p. 232-7.
142. Pulkkinen, L., et al., Mutations in the gamma 2 chain gene (LAMC2) of kalinin/laminin 5 in the junctional forms of epidermolysis bullosa. Nat Genet, 1994. 6(3): p. 293-7.
143. Baudoin, C., et al., A novel homozygous nonsense mutation in the LAMC2 gene in patients with the Herlitz junctional epidermolysis bullosa. Hum Mol Genet, 1994. 3(10): p.1909-10.
144. Aberdam, D., et al., Herlitz's junctional epidermolysis bullosa is linked to mutations in the gene (LAMC2) for the gamma 2 subunit of nicein/kalinin (LAMININ-5). Nat Genet, 1994. 6(3): p. 299-304.
145. McGrath, J.A., et al., Mutations in the 180-kD bullous pemphigoid antigen (BPAG2), a hemidesmosomal transmembrane collagen (COL17A1), in generalized atrophic benign epidermolysis bullosa. Nat Genet, 1995. 11(1): p. 83-6.

146. Pulkkinen, L., et al., Homozygous alpha6 integrin mutation in junctional epidermolysis bullosa with congenital duodenal atresia. Hum Mol Genet, 1997. 6(5): p. 669-74.
147. Ruzzi, L., et al., A homozygous mutation in the integrin alpha6 gene in junctional epidermolysis bullosa with pyloric atresia. J Clin Invest, 1997. 99(12): p. 2826-31.
148. Vidal, F., et al., Integrin beta 4 mutations associated with junctional epidermolysis bullosa with pyloric atresia. Nat Genet, 1995. 10(2): p. 229-34.
149. Koster, J., et al., Two different mutations in the cytoplasmic domain of the integrin beta 4 subunit in nonlethal forms of epidermolysis bullosa prevent interaction of beta 4 with plectin. J Invest Dermatol, 2001. 117(6): p. 1405-11.
150. Smith, F.J., et al., Plectin deficiency results in muscular dystrophy with epidermolysis bullosa. Nat Genet, 1996. 13(4): p. 450-7.
151. McLean, W.H., et al., Loss of plectin causes epidermolysis bullosa with muscular dystrophy: cDNA cloning and genomic organization. Genes Dev, 1996. 10(14): p. 1724-35.
152. Pulkkinen, L., et al., Homozygous deletion mutations in the plectin gene (PLEC1) in patients with epidermolysis bullosa simplex associated with late-onset muscular dystrophy. Hum Mol Genet, 1996. 5(10): p. 1539-46.
153. Chavanas, S., et al., A homozygous nonsense mutation in the PLEC1 gene in patients with epidermolysis bullosa simplex with muscular dystrophy. J Clin Invest, 1996. 98(10): p. 2196-200.
154. Weber, F., et al., Squamous cell carcinoma in junctional and dystrophic epidermolysis bullosa. Acta Derm Venereol, 2001. 81(3): p. 189-92.
155. Swensson, O. and Christophers, E. Generalized atrophic benign epidermolysis bullosa in 2 siblings complicated by multiple squamous cell carcinomas. Arch Dermatol, 1998. 134(2): p. 199-203.
156. Monk, B.E. and Pembroke, A.C. Epidermolysis bullosa with squamous cell carcinoma. Clin Exp Dermatol, 1987. 12(5): p. 373-4.
157. Mallipeddi, R., et al., Increased risk of squamous cell carcinoma in junctional epidermolysis bullosa. J Eur Acad Dermatol Venereol, 2004. 18(5): p. 521-6.
158. Lane, E.B., et al., A mutation in the conserved helix termination peptide of keratin 5 in hereditary skin blistering. Nature, 1992. 356(6366): p. 244-6.
159. Bonifas, J.M., Rothman, A.L. and Epstein, E.H. Jr., Epidermolysis bullosa simplex: evidence in two families for keratin gene abnormalities. Science, 1991. 254(5035): p. 1202-5.
160. Coulombe, P.A., et al., Point mutations in human keratin 14 genes of epidermolysis bullosa simplex patients: genetic and functional analyses. Cell, 1991. 66(6): p. 1301-11.
161. Ehrlich, P., et al., A common keratin 5 gene mutation in epidermolysis bullosa simplex-Weber-Cockayne. J Invest Dermatol, 1995. 104(5): p. 877-9.
162. Sasaki, Y., et al., A recurrent keratin 14 mutation in Dowling-Meara epidermolysis bullosa simplex. Br J Dermatol, 1999. 141(4): p. 747-8.
163. Ma, L., et al., A 'hot-spot' mutation alters the mechanical properties of keratin filament networks. Nat Cell Biol, 2001. 3(5): p. 503-6.
164. Shemanko, C.S., et al., Laryngeal involvement in the Dowling-Meara variant of epidermolysis bullosa simplex with keratin mutations of severely disruptive potential. Br J Dermatol, 2000. 142(2): p. 315-20.
165. Bernerd, F., et al., Clues to epidermal cancer proneness revealed by reconstruction of DNA repair-deficient xeroderma pigmentosum skin in vitro. Proc Natl Acad Sci U S A, 2001. 98(14): p. 7817-22.
166. Morykwas, M.J., et al., Growth and adherence of xeroderma pigmentosum keratinocytes in vitro. Ann Plast Surg, 1990. 24(4): p. 342-5.

Chapter 3

REGULATION OF CADHERINS DURING PROSTATE CANCER PROGRESSION

Ronald L. Heimark and Nelson R. Alexander
Department of Surgery and the Cancer Biology GraduateProgram, Arizona Health Sciences Center, University of Arizona, Tucson, AZ, USA

Abstract: Disruption of tight cell adhesion mediated by E-cadherin is an important step in carcinoma progression for cells to initiate cell migration and progress to metastasize. During prostate cacinogenesis, *E-cadherin* gene expression or function is downregulated through multiple mechanisms, many of which combine to silence *E-cadherin* expression through transcriptional regulation at the level of the *E-cadherin* promoter. Recent evidence indicates that concomitant with the transcriptional silencing of *E-cadherin* in prostate carcinomas, there is transcriptional upregulation of the mesenchymal cadherin, N-cadherin. The mechanisms of E- to N-cadherin switching in carcinomas and the potential roles of N-cadherin in tumor metastasis are summarized.

Key words: prostate cancer; metastasis; E-cadherin; N-cadherin; EMT; signaling

Integrity of epithelium lining the branching ductal network of the prostate gland is maintained through multiprotein adhesion complexes including tight junctions, adherens junctions, desmosomes and hemidesmosomes. The type 1 epithelial cadherin, E-cadherin, is a transmembrane protein that forms homotypic adhesive interactions at epithelial cell-cell adherens junctions. The E-cadherin cytoplasmic domain couples to catenins (α-, β-, γ-, and $p120^{ctn}$) and the actin cytoskeleton. The altered epithelial cytoarchitecture found in the progression of prostate adenocarcinomas is associated with a loss of integrin subunits and cadherin types, and with the gain of expression of different cadherin types (1). These changes disrupt tight epithelial cell-cell contacts and promote the release of invasive cells from the primary tumor.

A.E. Cress and R.B. Nagle (eds.), Cell Adhesion and Cytoskeletal Molecules in Metastasis, 47–67.

1. E-CADHERIN JUNCTIONS IN CANCER

Genetic and epigenetic alteration in E-cadherin/catenin function or gene expression is a central step in neoplastic process of metastasis of epithelial tumors from various tissues (2-4). This loss, in part, results in a transformation from the normal epithelial morphology toward a mesenchymal phenotype (5). This phenotype is reversed by transfection with full-length *E-cadherin* cDNA (6). Immunohistochemical analysis of highly invasive epithelial tumors (breast, melanoma, prostate) indicates that these tissues have decreased E-cadherin levels, suggesting a decreased function for E-cadherin in organization of tissue structure. Umbas et al. (7) found that human prostate carcinomas with a Gleason sum score >6 had decreased E-cadherin immunoreactivity compared to normal glandular epithelium, and tumors with a Gleason sum score of 9 had even lower E-cadherin immunoreactivity. In particular 63% of the tumors that extended beyond the prostate capsule, compared to 33% of organ confined tumors, had altered E-cadherin expression (8). Other studies evaluating E-cadherin expression and prostate cancer outcome have also demonstrated a correlation between decreased E-cadherin expression with increased prostate cancer grade (2-9). Decreased *E-cadherin* gene expression was found in microarray studies to correlate with comparison of prostate cancer and benign tissue (10). Moreover, the protocadherin *FAT*, which has been shown to have tumor suppressor functions, was also down regulated in metastatic prostate cancer. An apparent re-expression of E-cadherin in cell junctions has also been observed in metastatic tumor cells, and further suggests reversible epigenetic regulation of the cadherin/catenin complex (11).

The mechanisms underlying E-cadherin silencing in prostate cancer are not completely understood. The human *E-cadherin* gene (*CDH1*) is located on 16q22.1 and spans approximately 100 Kb (12). Genetic events such as mutations, loss of heterozygocity (LOH), and epigenetic regulation by transcriptional repression, and methylation of CpG islands in the promoter have been implicated in the regulation of *E-cadherin* gene. An important mechanism to silence *E-cadherin* expression *in vivo* is through methylation of CpG islands located within the 5'promoter of the *E-cadherin* gene. There are ~138 CpG islands in the *E-cadherin* gene spanning a 3000+ base pair region, from -1200 base pairs 5' to exon 2 (13). Epigenetic silencing by promoter methylation of CpG island on transcriptional repression of *E-cadherin* has been reported. Originally, hypermethylation of the CpG islands in the *E-cadherin* gene was reported in cell lines, including lines derived from prostate carcinoma, and correlated with transcriptional down regulation of the gene expression (14). In human prostate tumors, expression of *E-cadherin* is inactivated and the 5'promoter and first exon is methylated with varying prevalence (15-17). Methylation was found to occur in 30% of low grade microdissected prostate cancer samples In addition, methylation of the *CDH1* promoter is present in 70% of advanced prostate tumors (15).

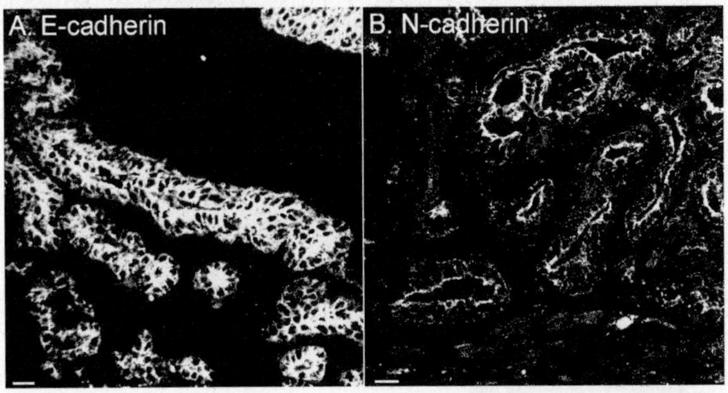

Figure 1. Indirect immunofluorescence analysis of expression of N-cadherin and E-cadherin in prostate cancer specimens. Frozen prostate tissues sections were immmunostained for E-cadherin and N-cadherin and grading was performed based on H & E-stained sections (data not shown). Images are of a grade 3 cancer and were contributed by Dr. R. Nagle. Note: staining of N-cadherin in both carcinoma cells and stromal cells.

2. ADHERIN SWITCHING DURING CANCER PROGRESSION

Several non-epithelial cadherin types, such as the type 1 neural cadherin, N-cadherin, and the type II cadherin, cadherin-11 (OB-cadherin), were found to be expressed in prostate carcinomas *in* vitro and *in vivo* (18-20). *In vitro* studies showed that inactivation of E-cadherin in prostate carcinoma cell lines is associated with the gain of expression of N-cadherin (20). N-cadherin is not expressed in normal adult prostatic epithelium, but is expressed in cells that surround the epithelium including smooth muscle, endothelium, and neurons (Figure 1). Prostate carcinoma cell lines in culture also show differential cadherin expression, displaying more than one type of cadherin. For example, the PC3 cell lines possess multiple cadherin types (19), notably cadherin–11, in addition to E-, and N-cadherin. N-cadherin expression can be detected in tumors with Gleason score above 7 (18, 20, 21). Stromal fibroblast cell lines from breast and prostate also express N-cadherin (20). In addition, N-cadherin promoted the heterotypic adhesive interaction of invasive prostate cancer cells with prostate stromal fibroblasts (20). These results suggest N-cadherin expression in carcinoma cells may promote their interaction with surrounding stromal cells, endothelial cells or neurons, thereby facilitating invasion and metastasis.

It has been suggested that unlike E-cadherin, N-cadherin and cadherin-11 promote motility and invasion of carcinoma cells (Figure 2). Over-expression of N-cadherin or cadherin-11 in E-cadherin expressing breast carcinoma cell line promotes cell migration and invasion (22-24). N-cadherin has been shown to promote cell motility and migration, as compared to the opposite effect of E-cadherin (22, 23, 25). N-cadherin-induced tumor cell invasion can even overcome E-cadherin mediated cell-cell adhesion (24, 26).

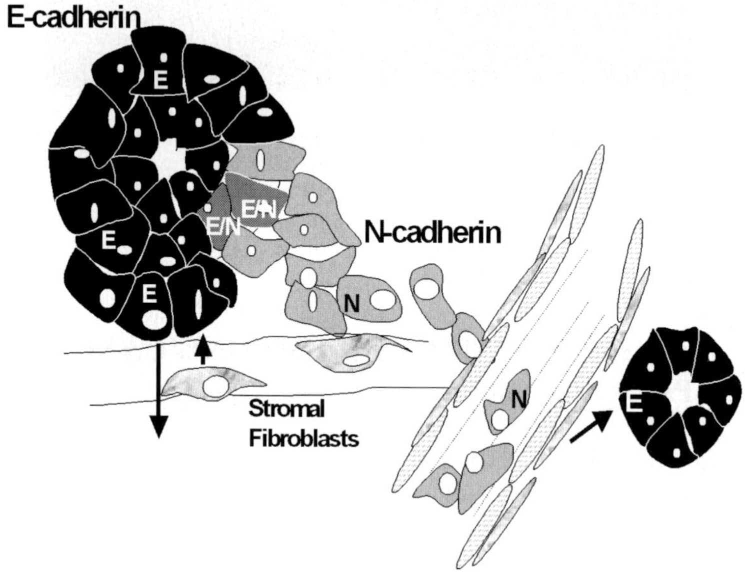

Figure 2. Schematic representation of transition of E-cadherin to N-cadherin during prostate tumor progression. Tumor cells expressing E-cadherin are shown in black and N-cadherin expression cells in gray. Prostate tumor cells express epithelial markers such as E-cadherin. The dynamics of cadherin expression in prostate caricnomas can be regulated by the tumor microenvironment. Induction of regulators such as Twist, ZEB1, Slug and Snail, repress E-cadherin gene expression in cancer cells. Mesenchymal markers, such as N-cadherin, are induced in these cancer cells. This leads to a less adhesive, more motile cell morphology that allows local invasion, intravasation into lymph or blood vessels and subseguent metastasis. At secondary sites, solitary carcinoma cells can extravasate and can form a new carcinoma expressing E-cadherin.

The phenotypic conversion from E-cadherin to N-cadherin expression in prostate carcinoma cells is a molecular alteration that is proposed to have dual functions. The switch facilitates tumor progression allowing cancer cells to detach from the primary tumor mass. In addition evidence suggests that during the transition from benign to invasive carcinoma the switch in cadherin types may support the malignant tumor phenotype and allow cells to survive and grow in ectopic sites (18). Expression of N-cadherin by prostate carcinoma cells lines correlates with invasion and suggests that invasion is mediated by N-cadherin-mediated interactions between the prostate cancer cells and stromal cells (20). The presence of N-cadherin in stromal cells surrounding glandular epithelium and in nerve bundles extending into the prostate could facilitate prostate carcinoma cell invasion, and extracapsular metastasis (27).

Epithelium can express more than one cadherin type as does endothelium (VE-cadherin and N-cadherin) and keratinocytes (E-cadherin and P-cadherin) (28-29). Different cadherins expressed in the same cells appear to directly affect each other's function. Suppression of N-cadherin function in invasive squamous carcinoma cells results in the induction of E-and P-cadherin expression and the reversion to an epithelial phenotype. In contrast, forced expression of N-cadherin in epithelial-like squamous cells causes downregulation of E- and P-cadherin and the acquisition of an invasive phenotype (22). This implies that the expression of N-cadherin during tumor progression might be necessary and sufficient to overcome E-cadherin-mediated cell-cell adhesion and to promote cancer progression. In high grade cancer specimens, Tomita et al. (18) showed that some carcinoma cells co-expressed both E- cadherin and N-cadherin. The prevailing model for regulation of E-cadherin and N-cadherin adhesion involves the catenins, since they functionally link the complex to the actin cytoskeleton. While E-cadherin functions to stabilize cell junctions (30), N-cadherin in association with the fibroblast growth factor receptor (FGFR) which promotes motile cell-cell contacts (31-33). The opposing functions of E-cadherin and N-cadherin in cell-cell adhesion and migration modulate cellular behavior. Evidence suggest that the role of N-cadherin is dominant in the processes of migration, invasion, and metastasis (20, 23, 26, 34). Steinberg and Takeichi (35) proposed that in a population of motile cohesive cells, such as a tumor, weaker cell attachments will be displaced by stronger ones, and cells will segregate into populations with the weaker population moving to the border of the mass. This hypothesis predicts that tumor cells expressing N-cadherin will separate from the tumor body and may for cell-cell contacts with N-cadherin expressing cells in the surrounding stroma.

3. MODULATION OF *E-CADHERIN* AND *N-CADHERIN* GENE EXPRESSION

While the causes of the perturbations of *E-cadherin* gene expression and function are not completely known, studies suggest that connections exist between integrin-mediated adhesion and signal transduction pathways, and imply a reversibility of epithelial cadherin gene expression (13). The 5'promoter of the *E-cadherin* gene *(CDH1)* is fundamental to the regulation of *E-cadherin* transcriptional activity. The mouse *E-cadherin* promoter was characterized by Behrens et al. (36), and has an a typical TATA box, a CCAAT box (-65 bp), a GC-rich region (-30 bp to -58 bp) and contains a palindromic region composed of two E-boxes (CACGTGCAGGTG). The transcription factors AP2 and SP1 bind to and drive the constitutive expression of *E-cadherin* in epithelium *in vitro* (37). Interestingly, Hennig et al. documented an epithelial-specific enhancer cis-element located within the first intron of the *E-cadherin* gene *in vitro* (37). While the mouse and human *E-cadherin* promoters display an extremely high degree of similarity, an additional fourth E-box element was found in the first intron of the human *E-cadherin* gene which is not present in mouse (38).

The E-boxes in the *E-cadherin* promoter have been shown to be important for transcriptional repression of E-*cadherin* during tumor progression. The major transcriptional repressor that has been shown to interact with these E-boxes is the zinc finger transcription factor family of Snail/Slug (39). Transcriptional repression of the human *E-cadherin* gene by Snail in *in vitro* studies has been shown to require the three E-boxes located in the 5'promoter of the human *E-cadherin* gene (39). These data strongly suggest that Snail is one of the major nuclear proteins that binds to the E-boxes within the 5'promoter of the *E-cadherin* gene and represses transcriptional activation. Recent studies also suggest that integrin-mediated adhesion through the downstream signaling of integrin-linked kinase (ILK) also plays a role in regulation of E-cadherin expression (40). The activation of integrin-linked kinase, which mediates signals from ECM increases expression of the zinc finger transcription factor Snail and downregulates *E-cadherin* (41). The Snail/Slug family proteins upregulate the transcriptional repressor ZEB1, which is also capable of binding to E-boxes in the promoter of *E-cadherin* and repressing transcription (42).

Other important transcriptional repressors of *E-cadherin* expression in tumor cells are E47, Slug, ZEB1(δEF1), and ZEB2 (42, 43). These transcription factors have also been shown to bind to the E-boxes located within the 5' promoter of *E-cadherin*. More recently, regulation of *E-cadherin* transcription by the bHLH Twist1 has proven to be an additional mechanism to down regulate the expression of *E-cadherin* (44). Twist1 has been shown to regulate metastasis of human breast cancer cells in a mouse orthotopic tumor model. *Twist* expression was shown not to contribute to cell proliferation or inhibition of apoptosis, in contrast Yang et al. (44) suggest that Twist may have a function unique to the induction of metastasis through the regulation of cell migration and invasion. In this work, inhibition of *Twist* gene expression with siRNA inhibited tumor metastasis *in vivo*, and overexpression of *mTwist* in breast epithelial cells upregulated mesenchymal markers such as fibronectin, vimentin and importantly N-cadherin. Concomitant with the upregulation of mesenchymal markers, epithelial genes such as *E-cadherin* were down regulated, and cell migration was increased *in vitro*. *Twist* mRNA was also shown to be upregulated in human breast cancer tissues by the expression of Wnt1, however gene expression of *E-cadherin* or *N-cadherin* was not examined (45).

Earlier work identified the bHLH factor Twist as a gene crucial for proper epithelial-to-mesenchymal transformation during gastrulation and mesoderm formation in *Drosophila* (46). The role of Twist factors across species is highly conserved exhibiting expression and function within mesoderm, muscle, bone, and limb development. Twist is also expressed in gastric cancer, and this expression correlated with *N-cadherin* gene expression (47). More recently, similar findings were found in prostate cancer tissues (48) where Twist expression correlated with increased Gleason score. Immunostaining of tumor sections for Twist detected both nuclear and cytoplasmic localization. Twist has been shown to interact with a number of other class A and class B bHLH proteins and also other transcription factor families. Twist has been shown to homodimerize, and heterodimerize with other bHLH proteins such as E12, Mef2 and MyoD in *Drosophila* and mice. The N-terminus of Twist was recently shown to interact with the homeobox transcription factor HOXA5 in breast tumorogenesis (49). The N-terminus of twist associates with other non bHLH transcription factors such as the histone acetyltransferases p300 and p300/CBP (50). Recent evidence suggests that phosphorylation of Twist1 in the HLH domain modulates the dimerization partner that Twist1 can bind (51). Together these data suggest that Twist is a potent transcriptional regulator of genes involved in the metastatic spread of carcinoma, including N-cadherin.

The *N-cadherin* gene *(CDH2)* was mapped to a 250 kb region on chromosome 18q11.2. and is composed of 16 exons (52). The 5'promoter of *N-cadherin* does not contain CCATT or typical TATA boxes, but does show a high GC content and several consensus Sp1 and AP2 binding sites (53). *N-cadherin* expression in osteoblasts has been shown to be regulated by SP1 and MZF-7 DNA binding sites between -161 bp and -131 bp in the 5'proximal promoter. This study defined the *N-cadherin* basal core promoter to be located between -335 bp and -18 bp in the 5'proximal promoter. The start of transcription is suggested to be at -42 bp 5' of the ATG start site. Whether Twist regulates *N-cadherin* gene expression directly or indirectly is unknown.

An early event in prostate carcinogenesis appears to be LOH of chromosome 8p, which occurs in approximately 80% of metastatic prostate cancers (54). The Nkx3.1 homeobox gene, located on chromosome 8p21, is a candidate for a prostate specific tumor suppressor since conditional loss of Nkx3.1 in adult mice has been shown to induce PIN lesions (55). LOH at chromosome 10q is frequently associated with advanced prostate cancer(56). The *PTEN* gene located on chromosome 10q23 encodes a lipid phosphatase that negatively regulates phosphatidylinositol 3'-kinase (PI 3-kinase)/Akt signaling pathway. Haploinsufficiency of PTEN+/-; Nkx3.1+/- mice over 1 year were shown to develop invasive cancer with heterogeneous E-cadherin expression (57). While the role of Nkx3.1 in *E-cadherin* regulation is not clear, the PI 3-kinase/PTEN/AKT signaling pathway can inactivate the glycogen synthase kinase 3β and stabilize the protein degradation of Snail and by activating transcription of *Snail* (58, 59).

4. CONSEQUENCES OF E-CADHERIN TO N-CADHERIN SWITCHING

Several signaling proteins interact either directly with the cadherin cytoplasmic domain or with the catenins and are possible regulators of cadherin function. The $p120^{ctn}$ binds to the cadherin juxtamembrane region and is implicated in cadherin cis-interactions to form homodimers. The strength of cadherin adhesion and stability in the membrane controls cell motility(30, 60). The functional role of $p120^{ctn}$, originally identified as a Src kinase substrate, in regulating cadherin adhesion is probably through phosphorylation. $p120^{ctn}$ tyrosine phosphorylation is elevated in cell junctions suggesting that it may function in junction maturation. Over expression of $p120^{ctn}$ in epithelium induces a more motile mesenchymal phenotype through inhibition of RhoA GTPase by $p120^{ctn}$ maintaining RhoA in the inactive GDP state (61, 62) and enhanced lamellapodia formation (62). RhoA was previously shown to be involved in cadherin clustering through the mobilization of actin to sites if cell-cell contact (63, 64).

The adhesive properties of cadherins are regulated by the activities of the Rho family of GTPases, which remodels the actin cytoskeleton. Expression of constitutively active Rac1, or a guanine exchange factor for Rac1, Tiam1, increases the adhesive activity of E-cadherin (63, 64). CDC42 and Rac1 have been shown to regulate E-cadherin activity through the activity of

IQGAP. IQGAP seems to bind directly to and inhibit the cadherin association with actin through α-catenin. Active CDC42 and Rac1 inhibit the ability of IQGAP to bind β-catenin, thereby maintaining cadherin adhesion (65). The effects of RhoA on E-cadherin activity are less consistent. This could be due to more recent findings that the activity of RhoA is inhibited following the ligation of E-cadherin (62). This suggests that the activity of E-cadherin requires the precise regulation of RhoA activity. Both Rac1 and RhoA are necessary to initiate E-cadherin adhesion; Rac1 may be required to maintain the cadherin/catenin linkage to the cytoskeleton, and the continuous activity of RhoA may inhibit Rac1 activity (66).

β-catenin binds α-catenin, an actin binding protein, which then links directly to the actin cytoskeleton, and has an essential role in the structural organization of adherens junctions. Serine/threonine phosphorylation of β-catenin or E-cadherin results in the stabilization of the cadherin/catenin complex. Evidence indicates that migration of epithelial cells is associated with increased tyrosine phosphorylation of β-catenin (67). One of the non-receptor tyrosine kinases that has been shown to phosphorylate β-catenin is Fer kinase(fes-related protein), which also phoshorylates $p120^{ctn}$ and cortactin (68). Phosphorylated β-catenin on tyrosine 142 correlated with inhibition of cadherin-mediated adhesion and adhesion of α-catenin to β-catenin (69). Fer kinase is expressed in prostate carcinoma cell lines and reduction of Fer kinase expression by antisense reduces cell proliferation (70). Fer kinase has been identified in N-cadherin/catenin complexes and binds to β-catenin and $p120^{ctn}$ binds through interaction with the coiled coil domain of p120. Evidence also suggests that cross-talk between N-cadherin and β1 integrins is mediated by Fer kinase (71).

Fer kinase has been shown to bind to both β1 integrins and N-cadherin/catenin complexes. Inhibition of the association between N-cadherin and Fer inhibits the phosphorylation of p130cas (71). This activity may be dependent on Fer mediated sequestration of phosphatases, such that when Fer is associated with integrin adhesion structures, it recruits a phosphatase, possibly PTP1B or PTP-PEST, which inactivates p130cas. PTP1B associates with N-cadherin at a domain that partially overlaps with the β-catenin binding domain. The interaction of N-cadherin with PTP1B is essential for its association with β-catenin, which is critical to cadherin adhesive function. A class of heterotrimeric G proteins, Gα12/13 also associates with the cytoplasmic domain of N-cadherin. The cadherin binding site for Gα12/13 overlaps the PTP1B and can displace PTP1B from the cadherin complex (72, 73). Gα12/13 functions in the activation of Rho GTPase and its downstream effectors and may regulate cadherin function (74).

In addition to PTP1B, the phosphatases, PTPK, PTPμ, PTP-LAR, PCP-2, DEP-1 and Shp-2 reside in adherens junctions associated with cadherins(75-79). Re-expression of PTPμ in LNCaP prostate carcinoma cells that have weak E-cadherin adhesion restores strong cell-cell adhesion through regulation RACK1 , a receptor for activated protein kinase C (80,81). This association in adherens junctions suggests that regulating phosphorylation of cadherins and associated proteins may provide a rapid means for modulation of cell-cell adhesion.

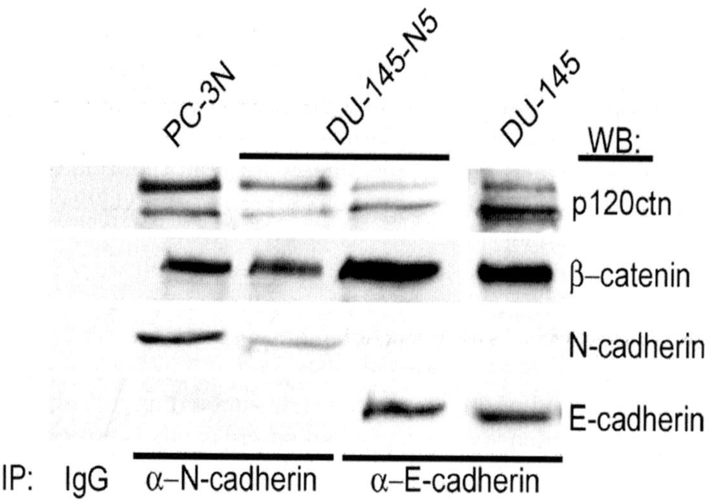

Figure 3. Analysis of p120^{ctn} isoforms and β-catenin associated with N- and E-cadherin from clone DU145-N5. As control, N-cadherin was immunoprecipitated from PC-3N, while E-cadherin was immunoprecipitated from DU145. Immmunoprecipitation of E- and N-cadherin was followed by immunoblot analysis for E-and N-cadherin, p120^{ctn} and β-catenin.

Since E-cadherin and N-cadherin were found to be co-expressed in cells of high grade prostate cancer tissue, we examined the effect of N-cadherin mis-expression on an E-cadherin positive prostate carcinoma line DU145. To evaluate the effect of co-expression of E and N-cadherin on the migratory phenotype, an N-cadherin/GFP fusion construct was transfected into DU145 prostate carcinoma cells. Clones expressing the N-cadherin/GFP or GFP empty vector were isolated through serial dilution, and selected under antibiotic resistance (82).

After selection of clonal cell lines, they were characterized for protein levels of E-cadherin, N-cadherin, p120^{ctn} and β-catenin. The clones showed variable levels of E-cadherin expression, but β-catenin appeared to be unchanged. The N-cadherin DU145 clone 5 (DU145-N5) showed lower levels of E-cadherin than N-cadherin, therefore we characterized this clone further. The presence of N-cadherin in DU145 cells increases the level of the $p120^{ctn1}$ isoform compared with the $p120^{ctn3}$ isoform in cellular lysates of DU145 cells. Analysis of the $p120^{ctn}$ isoforms by immunoprecipitation and immunoblotting showed that in DU145-N5 cells, there also appears to be preferential cadherin binding of $p120^{ctn1}$ vs. $p120^{ctn3}$ in lysates immunoprecipitated with either E-cadherin or N-cadherin antibodies. Preferential binding of the $p120^{ctn1}$ isoform with N-cadherin, and $p12^{ctn3}$ isoform binding with E-cadherin was found in the adhesion complexes (Figure 3). There are four $p120^{ctn1-4}$ isoforms arising from alternative splicing (83). The $p120^{ctn1}$ isoform contains an N-terminal coiled-coil domain and is preferentially expressed in motile cells. Epithelial cells preferentially express the $p120^{ctn3}$ isoform, which lacks the coiled-coil domain and supports cadherin stability and adhesion (84). Figure 4A shows that the peripheral actin cytoskeleton in clone 5, which is mis-expressing N-cadherin, is less well developed and that E-cadherin junctional localization is discontinuous. There is also more cell surface labeling of E-cadherin in a punctate distribution.

To analyze the functional consequences of mis-expression of N-cadherin in DU145 cells, we determined the rates of cell migration. Cells were plated at confluent density overnight in serum-free media and a linear migration assay was performed according to the method of Berens et al. (85). We selected this assay because cells initially form a contiguous monolayer before migration is initiated. Quantitation of the migration difference showed that clone 5 mis-expressing N-cadherin had nearly 2.6 times the migration rate of the parental DU145 (Figure 4B). Vinculin localization showed reduced incorporation in lamellipodia in N-cadherin/DU145 cells even though they display more lamellipodia than DU145. As a whole, the literature concerning N-cadherin function strongly indicates that N-cadherin expression is an important mediator of the mesenchymal phenotype (86). Accordingly, forced N-cadherin expression in epithelial tumor cells induces a migratory phenotype which is dominant over the ability of E-cadherin to repress migration (22, 26).

The functional implications of the change from E-cadherin to N-cadherin for tumor progression suggest potential roles beyond cell detachment in promoting metastasis. During gastrulation, the E- to N-cadherin switch permits the segregation of mesoderm from ectoderm and endoderm. Unlike

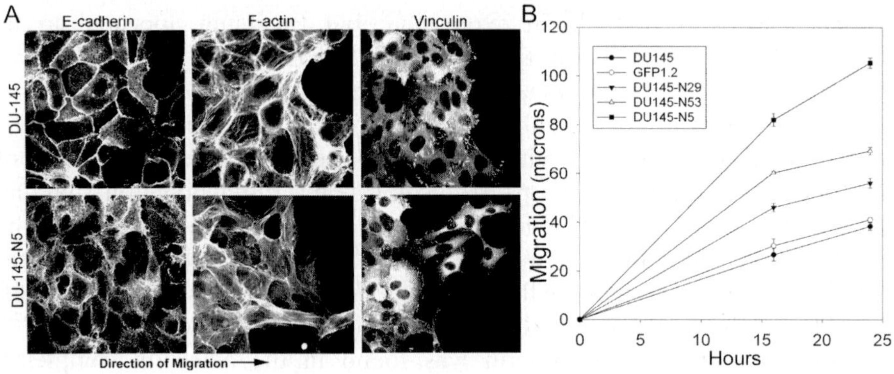

Figure 4A/4B. Co-expression of E-cadherin and N-cadherin induces cell migration in prostate carcinoma cells. (A). Localizatin of the F-actin, vinculin and E-cadherin in DU145 and DU145-N5 at the migrating leading edge. Immunofluorescence of F-actin was carried out using rhodamine phalloidin, while for E-cadherin and vinculin, was carried out using Mabs. Cells were plated on Laminin-1 coated slides. (B) Time course of cell migration. Cells were plated at confluent density. Values are means of 3 independent experiments. The migration of three N-cadherinGFP clones (DU145-N5, DU145-N29, DU145-N53) are compared to DU145 cells and a DU145 clone expressing GFP (GFP1.2). DU145-N5 showed the highest rate of migration.

E-cadherin, N-cadherin and cadherin-11 promote a dynamic adhesion state. N-cadherin mediated neurite outgrown and cell migration is inhibited by inhibitors of the fibroblast growth factor receptor (FGFR), and extracellular portions of the two proteins interact (32, 87). N-cadherin may be involved in both ligand dependent and independent activation of the FGFR. The cis-interactions of N-cadherin molecules associated with the FGFR may bring the kinase domains of the FGFR in close enough proximity to induce cross-phosphorylation. Conversely, it has been shown in breast cancer cells that N-cadherin stabilizes the FGFR and inhibits the internalization of the receptor, thereby enhancing activation potential (32). The HAV sequence in FGFR associates with the fourth extracellular domain of N-cadherin (87). Although N-cadherin cooperation with the FGFR certainly has the potential to induce cell migration and cancer cell invasion through FGFR signaling alone, many of the signaling partners with the FGFR, specifically tyrosine kinases like Src and tyrosine phosphatases like PTP1B, associate with and regulate the activity of the β1 integrin. During cell migration cross-talk between β1 integrin and cadherins has been demonstrated to regulate cadherin junctional adhesion (71, 88-90).

5. CONCLUSION

Prostate cancer mortality typically results from metastasis to lymph nodes and bone and progression from androgen-dependent to androgen-independent growth. Evidence suggests that progression of carcinomas, in part, results from the acquisition of resistance to apoptosis (91). Switching from E-cadherin to N-cadherin activates expression of the anti-apoptotic protein bcl-2 through signaling of PI 3-kinase and actin cytoskeletal reorganization (92). The switching of cadherin types suggests transformation of epithelium-to-mesenchyme (EMT) during tumor progression mediates local invasion and metastasis. The silencing of *E-cadherin* gene expression is an important step in EMT which increases tumor cell invasiveness through detachment of cells from the tumor mass. Since the inhibition of E-cadherin can occur through both reversible and irreversible mechanisms, this suggests that EMT may follow a similar pattern. Evidence shows that the decreased expression of E-cadherin in prostate tumors correlates with higher Gleason scores characteristic of less differentiated more aggressive tumors (8). The process of EMT also results in the acquisition of mesenchymal characteristics by carcinoma cells, such as the gain of N-cadherin. It is thought that at any one time, EMT may occur in only a subpopulation of tumor cells during prostate tumor metastasis. Since the process of metastasis has been shown to be very inefficient in xenograft models, the gain of N-cadherin may appears to promote cell survival through the activation of PKB/Akt.

N-cadherin ligation has been shown to activate the PI 3-kinase signaling cascade, in addition to activating Rac1 GTPase (92, 93). A balance between the activation of Rac1, CDC42 and RhoA determine the cellular phenotype and motility by regulation of actin cytoskeleton remodeling. The direct ligation of N-cadherin cell adhesion, both through calcium switch and antibody activation assays, induces the association of the p85 subunit of the PI 3-kinase with the cytoplasmic domain of N-cadherin (92). This recruitment or PI 3-kinase to the adherens junction complex required an intact actin cytoskeleton. This then activates the PKB/Akt pathway, which inactivates the pro-apoptotic molecule Bad and increases the anti-apoptotic protein bcl-2. Increased Akt kinase activity has been suggested to function in the progression of prostate cancer. Over expression of activated Akt was sufficient to facilitate increased tumor growth in a murine xenograft model and over expression is sufficient in transgenic mouse model to induce prostatic intraepithelial neoplasia (94). Activated Akt is increased in high Gleason grade prostate cancer and was found to be a significant predictor of poor outcome (95). Increased bcl-2 levels in prostate carcinomas strongly correlates with the recurrence of disease and progression to androgen-independent growth (96-98). Moreover, over-expression of the human bcl-2 transgene with a prostate specific promoter mediates resistance to apoptosis of glandular epithelium induced by androgen withdrawal (99). N-cadherin signaling activates both the Rac GTPase and the PI 3-kinase signal transduction pathways are important for tumor cell survival and migration and contribute to metastasis.

One of the hallmarks of metastatic carcinoma is the down regulation of *E-cadherin*, either at the level of function or gene expression. In prostate carcinomas that had silenced *E-cadherin* transcription, *N-cadherin* expression was detected. However, rather than simply mediating cell:cell adhesion in tumor cells, evidence demonstrates the ability of N-cadherin to serve as an initiator of intracellular signaling, activating distinct pathways from E-cadherin. Genetic analysis of the function of E- and N-cadherin *in vitro* and *in vivo* clearly indicates that these two cadherins are required for development, and have non-redundant functional roles in cellular differentiation. The acquisition of N-cadherin by migrating carcinoma cells supports their interaction with cells of the surrounding stroma, including myofibroblasts, neurons and endothelium. Signaling pathways activated by stromal-carcinoma adhesions can support survival and migration of carcinoma cells in tumor progression.

ACKNOWLEDGEMENTS

This work was supported by NIH grant PO1 CA 56666.

REFERENCES

1. Nagle, R.B., Knox, J.D., Wolf, C., Bowden, G.T., and Cress, A.E., 1994, Adhesion molecules, extracellular matrix, and proteases in prostate carcinoma, J. Cellular Biochem. 19: 232-237.
2. Ross, J.S., Figge, H.L., Bui, H.X., del Rosario, A.D., Fisher, H.A., Nazeer, T.X., Ingle, R., and Kim, D.N., 1994, E-cadherin expression in prostatic carcinoma biopsies: correlation with tumor grade, DNA content, pathologic stage, and clinical outcome, Modern Pathology 7: 835-841.
3. Schipper, J.H., Frixen, U.H., Behrens, J., Unger, A., Jahnke, K., and Birchmeier, W., 1991, E-cadherin expression in squamous cell carcinomas of head and neck: inverse correlation with tumor dedifferentiation and lymph node metastasis. Cancer Res. 51: 6328-6337.
4. Moll, R., Mitze, M., Frixen, U.H., and Birchmeier, W., 1993, Differential loss of E-cadherin expression in infiltrating ductal and lobular breast carcinomas. Am. J. Pathol. 143: 1731-1742.

5. Behrens, J., Mareel, M.M., Van Roy, F.M., and Birchmeier, W., 1989, Dissecting tumor cell invasion: epithelial cells acquire invasive properties after the loss of uvomorulin-mediated cell- cell adhesion. J. Cell Biol. 108: 2435-2447.
6. Nagafuchi, A., Takeichi, M., 1988, Cell binding function of E-cadherin is regulated by the cytoplasmic domain. EMBO J. 7: 3679-3684.
7. Umbas, R., Schalken, J.A., Aalders, T.W., Carter, B.S., Karthaus, H.F., Schaafsma, H.E., and Isaacs, W.B., 1992, Expression of the cellular adhesion molecule E-cadherin is reduced or absent in high-grade prostate cancer. Cancer Res. 52: 5104-5109.
8. Umbas, R., Isaacs, W.B., Bringuier, P.P., Schaafsma, H.E., Karthaus, H.F., Oosterhof, G.O., Debruyne, F.M., and Schalken, J.A., 1994, Decreased E-cadherin expression is associated with poor prognosis in patients with prostate cancer. Cancer Res. 54: 3929-3933.
9. Kuczyk, M., Serth, J., Machtens, S., Bokemeyer, C., Bathke, W., Stief, C., and Jonas, U., 1998, Expression of E-cadherin in primary prostate cancer: correlation with clinical features, Br. J. Urol. 81: 406-412.
10. Dhanasekaran, S.M., Barrette, T.R., Ghosh, D., Shah, R., Varambally, S., Kurachi, K., Pienta, K.J., Rubin, M.A., and Chinnaiyan, A.M., 2001, Delineation of prognostic biomarkers in prostate cancer. Nature 412: 822-826.
11. De Marzo, A.M., Knudsen, B., Chan-Tack, K., and Epstein, J.I., 1999, E-cadherin expression as a marker of tumor aggressiveness in routinely processed radical prostatectomy specimens, Urology 53: 707-713.
12. Berx, G., Staes, K., van Hengel, J., Molemans, F., Bussemakers, M.J., van Bokhoven, A., and Van Roy, F., 1995, Cloning and characterization of the human invasion suppressor gene E-cadherin (CDH1). Genomics 26: 281-289.
13. Graff, J.R., Gabrielson, E., Fujii, H., Baylin, S.B., and Herman, J.G., 2000, Methylation patterns of the E-cadherin 5' CpG island are unstable and reflect the dynamic, heterogeneous loss of E-cadherin expression during metastatic progression. J. Biol. Chem. 275: 2727-2732.
14. Graff, J.R., Herman, J.G., Lapidus, R.G., Chopra, H., Xu, R., Jarrard, D.F. X.I. W., Pitha, P.M., Davidson, N.E., and Baylin, S.B., 1995, E-cadherin expression is silenced by DNA hypermethylation in human breast and prostate carcinomas. Cancer Res. 55: 5195-5199.
15. Li, L.C., Zhao, H., Nakajima, K., Oh, B.R., Ribeiro Filho, L.A., Carroll, P., and Dahiya, R, 2001, Methylation of the E-cadherin gene promoter correlates with progression of prostate cancer. J. Urol. 166: 705-709.
16. Kallakury, B.V., Sheehan, C.E., Winn-Deen, E., Oliver, J., Fisher, H.A., Kaufman, R.P., Jr., and Ross, J.S., 2001, Decreased expression of catenins (alpha and beta), p120 CTN, and E-cadherin cell adhesion proteins and E-cadherin gene promoter methylation in prostatic adenocarcinomas. Cancer 92: 2786-2795.
17. Kang, G.H., Lee, S., Lee, H.J., and Hwang, K.S., 2004, Aberrant CpG island hypermethylation of multiple genes in prostate cancer and prostatic intraepithelial neoplasia. J. Pathol. 202: 233-240.
18. Tomita, K., van Bokhoven, A., van Leenders, G.J., Ruijter, E.T., Jansen, C.F., Bussemakers, M.J., and Schalken, J.A., 2000, Cadherin switching in human prostate cancer progression. Cancer Res. 60: 3650-3654.
19. Bussemakers, M.J., van Bokhoven, A., Tomita, K., Jansen, C.F., and Schalken, J.A., 2000, Complex cadherin expression in human prostate cancer cells. Int. J. Cancer 85: 446-450.

20. Tran, N.L., Cress, A.E., Nagle, R.B., and Heimark, R.L., 1999, Expression of N-cadherin in Invasive Human Prostate Carcinomas: Transformation from an Epithelial to a Mesenchymal Phenotype. Am. J. Pathol. 155: 787-798.
21. Jaggi, M., Nazemi, T., Abrahams, N.A., Baker, J.J., Galich, A., Smith, L.M., and Balaji, K.C., 2005, N-cadherin switching occurs in high Gleason grade prostate cancer. Prostate.
22. Islam, S., Carey, T.E., Wolf, G.T., Wheelock, M.J., and Johnson, K.R., 1996, Expression of N-cadherin by human squamous carcinoma cells induces a scattered fibroblastic phenotype with disrupted cell-cell adhesion. J. of Cell Biol. 135: 1643-1654.
23. Hazan, R.B., Kang, L., Whooley, B.P., and Borgen, P.I., 1997, N-cadherin promotes adhesion between invasive breast cancer cells and the stroma. Cell Adhesion & Communication 4: 399-411.
24. Nieman, M.T., Prudoff, R.S., Johnson, K.R., and Wheelock, M.J., 1999, N-cadherin promotes motility in human breast cancer cells regardless of their E-cadherin expression. J. Cell Biol. 147: 631-644.
25. Li, Y., Liu, W., Hayward, S.W., Cunha, G.R., and Baskin, L.S., 2000, Plasticity of the urothelial phenotype: effects of gastro-intestinal mesenchyme/stroma and implications for urinary tract reconstruction. Differentiation 66: 126-135.
26. Hazan, R.B., Phillips, G.R., Qiao, R.F., Norton, L., and Aaronson, S.A., 2000, Exogenous expression of N-cadherin in breast cancer cells induces cell migration, invasion, and metastasis. J. Cell Biol. 148: 779-790.
27. Villers, A., McNeal, J.E., Redwine, E.A., Freiha, F.S., and Stamey, T.A., 1989, The role of perineural space invasion in the local spread of prostatic adenocarcinoma. J. Urology 142: 763-768.
28. Navarro, P., Ruco, L., and Dejana, E., 1998, Differential localization of VE- and N-cadherins in human endothelial cells: VE-cadherin competes with N-cadherin for junctional localization. J. of Cell Biol. 140: 1475-1484.
29. Johnson, K.R., Lewis, J.E., Li, D., Wahl, J., Soler, A.P., Knudsen, K.A., Wheelock, and M.J., 1993, P- and E-cadherin are in separate complexes in cells expressing both cadherins. Exp. Cell Res. 207: 252-260.
30. Chen, H., Paradies, N.E., Fedor-Chaiken, M., and Brackenbury, R., 1997, E-cadherin mediates adhesion and suppresses cell motility via distinct mechanisms. J. Cell Science 110: 345-356.
31. Williams, E.J., Furness, J., Walsh, F.S., and Doherty, P., 1994, Activation of the FGF receptor underlies neurite outgrowth stimulated by L1, N-CAM, and N-cadherin. Neuron 13: 583-594.
32. Suyama, K., Shapiro, I., Guttman, M., and Hazan, R.B., 2002, A signaling pathway leading to metastasis is controlled by N-cadherin and the FGF receptor. Cancer Cell 2: 301-314.
33. Kim, J.B., Islam, S., Kim, Y.J., Prudoff, R.S., Sass, K.M., Wheelock, MJ, and Johnson, K.R., 2000, N-Cadherin extracellular repeat 4 mediates epithelial to mesenchymal transition and increased motility. J. Cell Biol. 151: 1193-1206.
34. Luo, Y., Radice, G.L., 2005, N-cadherin acts upstream of VE-cadherin in controlling vascular morphogenesis. J. Cell Biol. 169: 29-34.
35. Steinberg, M.S., Takeichi, M., 1994, Experimental specification of cell sorting, tissue spreading, and specific spatial patterning by quantitative differences in cadherin expression. Proc. Natl. Acad. Sci. USA, 91: 206-209.
36. Behrens, J., Lowrick, O., Klein-Hitpass, L., and Birchmeier, W., 1991, The E-cadherin promoter: functional analysis of a G.C-rich region and an epithelial cell-specific palindromic regulatory element. Proc. Natl. Acad. Sci. USA, 88: 11495-11499.

37. Hennig, G., Lowrick, O., Birchmeier, W., and Behrens, J., 1996, Mechanisms identified in the transcriptional control of epithelial gene expression. J. Biol. Chem. 271: 595-602.
38. Comijn, J., Berx, G., Vermassen, P., Verschueren, K., van Grunsven, L., Bruyneel, E., Mareel, M., Huylebroeck, D., and Van Roy, F., 2001, The two-handed E box binding zinc finger protein SIP1 downregulates E-cadherin and induces invasion. Mol. Cell 7: 1267-1278.
39. Batlle, E., Sancho, E., Franci, C., Dominguez, D., Monfar, M., Baulida, J., and Garcia, d. H., 2000, The transcription factor snail is a repressor of E-cadherin gene expression in epithelial tumour cells. Nature Cell Biology 2: 84-89.
40. Novak, A., Hsu, S.C., Leung-Hagesteijn, C., Radeva, G., Papkoff, J., Montesano, R., Roskelley, C., Grosschedl, R., and Dedhar, S., 1998, Cell adhesion and the integrin-linked kinase regulate the LEF-1 and beta-catenin signaling pathways. Proc. Natl. Acad. Sci. USA, 95, 4374-4379.
41. Tan, C., Costello, P., Sanghera, J., Dominguez, D., Baulida, J., de Herreros, A.G., and Dedhar, S., 2001, Inhibition of integrin linked kinase (ILK) suppresses beta-catenin-Lef/Tcf-dependent transcription and expression of the E-cadherin repressor, snail, in APC-/- human colon carcinoma cells. Oncogene, 20 133-140.
42. Guaita, S., Puig, I., Franci, C., Garrido, M., Dominguez, D., Batlle, E., Sancho, E., Dedhar, S., de Herreros, A.G., and Baulida, J., 2002, Snail induction of epithelial to mesenchymal transition in tumor cells is accompanied by MUC1 repression and ZEB1 expression . J. Biol. Chem. 277: 39209-39216.
43. Perez-Moreno, M.A., Locascio, A., Rodrigo, I., Dhondt, G., Portillo, F., Nieto, M.A., and Cano, A., 2001, A new role for E12/E47 in the repression of E-cadherin expression and epithelial-mesenchymal transitions. J. Biol. Chem. 276: 27424-27431.
44. Yang, J., Mani, S.A., Donaher, J.L., Ramaswamy, S., Itzykson, R.A., Come, C., Savagner, P., Gitelman, I., Richardson, A., and Weinberg, R.A., 2004, Twist, a master regulator of morphogenesis, plays an essential role in tumor metastasis. Cell 117: 927-939.
45. Howe, L.R., Watanabe, O., Leonard, J., and Brown, A.M., 2003, Twist is up-regulated in response to Wnt1 and inhibits mouse mammary cell differentiation. Cancer Res. 63: 1906-1913.
46. Oda, H., Tsukita, S., and Takeichi, M., 1998, Dynamic behavior of the cadherin-based cell-cell adhesion system during Drosophila gastrulation. Dev. Biol. 203: 435-450.
47. Rosivatz, E., Becker, I., Specht, K., Fricke, E., Luber, B., Busch, R., Hofler, H., and Becker, K.F., 2002, Differential expression of the epithelial-mesenchymal transition regulators snail, SIP1, and twist in gastric cancer. Am. J. Pathol. 161: 1881-1891.
48. Kwok, W.K., Ling, M.T., Lee, T.W., Lau, T.C., Zhou, C., Zhang, X., Chua, C.W., Chan, K.W., Chan, F.L., Glackin, C., Wong, Y.C., and Wang, X., 2005, Up-regulation of TWIST in prostate cancer and its implication as a therapeutic target. Cancer Res. 65: 5153-5162.
49. Stasinopoulos, I.A., Mironchik, Y., Raman, A., Wildes, F., Winnard, P., Jr., and Raman, V., 2005, HOXA5-twist interaction alters p53 homeostasis in breast cancer cells. J. Biol. Chem., 280: 2294-2299.
50. Hamamori, Y., Sartorelli, V., Ogryzko, V., Puri, P.L., Wu, H.Y., Wang, J.Y., Nakatani, Y., and Kedes, L., 1999, Regulation of histone acetyltransferases p300 and PCAF by the bHLH protein twist and adenoviral oncoprotein E1A. Cell 96: 405-413.
51. Firulli, B.A., Krawchuk, D., Centonze, V.E., Vargesson, N., Virshup, D.M., Conway, S.J., Cserjesi, P., Laufer, E., and Firulli, A.B., 2005, Altered Twist1 and Hand2

dimerization is associated with Saethre-Chotzen syndrome and limb abnormalities. Nat.Genet. 37: 373-381.

52. Wallis, J., Fox, M.F., and Walsh, F.S., 1994, Structure of the human N-cadherin gene: YAC analysis and fine chromosomal mapping to 18q11.2. Genomics 22: 172-179.
53. Le Mee, S., Fromigue, O., and Marie, P.J., 2005, Sp1/Sp3 and the myeloid zinc finger gene MZF1 regulate the human N-cadherin promoter in osteoblasts. Exp.Cell Res. 302: 129-142.
54. Bowen, C., Bubendorf, L., Voeller, H.J., Slack, R., Willi, N., Sauter, G., Gasser, T.C., Koivisto, P., Lack, E.E., Kononen, J., Kallioniemi, O.P., and Gelmann, E.P., 2000, Loss of NKX3.1 expression in human prostate cancers correlates with tumor progression. Cancer Res. 60: 6111-6115.
55. Abdulkadir, S.A., Magee, J.A., Peters, T.J., Kaleem, Z., Naughton, C.K., Humphrey, P.A., and Milbrandt, J., 2002, Conditional loss of Nkx3.1 in adult mice induces prostatic intraepithelial neoplasia . Mol. Cell Biol. 22: 1495-1503.
56. Li, J., Yen, C., Liaw, D., Podsypanina, K., Bose, S., Wang, S.I., Puc, J., Miliaresis, C., Rodgers, L., McCombie, R., Bigner, S.H., Giovanella, B.C., Ittmann, M., Tycko, B., Hibshoosh, H., Wigler, M.H., and Parsons, R., 1997, PTEN, a putative protein tyrosine phosphatase gene mutated in human brain, breast, and prostate cancer. Science, 275, 1943-1947.
57. Abate-Shen, C., Banach-Petrosky, W.A., Sun, X., Economides, K.D., Desai, N., Gregg, J.P., Borowsky, A.D., Cardiff, R.D., and Shen, M.M., 2003, Nkx3.1; Pten mutant mice develop invasive prostate adenocarcinoma and lymph node metastases. Cancer Research.63:3886-90.
58. Bachelder, R.E., Yoon, S.O., Franci, C., de Herreros, A.G., and Mercurio, A.M., 2005, Glycogen synthase kinase-3 is an endogenous inhibitor of Snail transcription: implications for the epithelial-mesenchymal transition . J. Cell Biol. 168: 29-33.
59. Zhou, B.P., Deng, J., Xia, W., Xu, J., Li, Y.M., Gunduz, M., and Hung, M.C., 2004, Dual regulation of Snail by GSK-3beta-mediated phosphorylation in control of epithelial-mesenchymal transition. Nat. Cell Biol., 6: 931-940.
60. Yap, A.S., Niessen, C.M., and Gumbiner, B.M., 1998, The juxtamembrane region of the cadherin cytoplasmic tail supports lateral clustering, adhesive strengthening, and interaction with p120ctn. J. Cell Biol. 141: 779-789.
61. Anastasiadis, P.Z., Moon, S.Y., Thoreson, M.A., Mariner, D.J., Crawford, H.C., Zheng, Y., and Reynolds, A.B., 2000, Inhibition of RhoA by p120 catenin. Nature Cell Biology 2: 637-644.
62. Noren, N.K., Liu, B.P., Burridge, K., and Kreft, B., 2000, p120 catenin regulates the actin cytoskeleton via Rho family GTPases. J. Cell Biol. 150: 567-580.
63. Braga, V.M., Machesky, L.M., Hall, A., and Hotchin, N.A., 1997, The small GTPases Rho and Rac are required for the establishment of cadherin-dependent cell-cell contacts. J. Cell Biol. 137: 1421-1431.
64. Takaishi, K., Sasaki, T., Kotani, H., Nishioka, H., and Takai, Y., 1997, Regulation of cell-cell adhesion by rac and rho small G proteins in MDCK cells. J. Cell Biol. 139: 1047-1059.
65. Kuroda, S., Fukata, M., Nakagawa, M., Fujii, K., Nakamura, T., Ookubo, T., Izawa, I., Nagase, T., Nomura, N., Tani, H., Shoji, I., Matsuura, Y., Yonehara, S., and Kaibuchi, K., 1998, Role of IQGAP1, a target of the small GTPases Cdc42 and Rac1, in regulation of E-cadherin- mediated cell-cell adhesion. Science 281: 832-835.

66. Malliri, A., van Es, S., Huveneers, S., and Collard, J.G., 2004, The Rac exchange factor Tiam1 is required for the establishment and maintenance of cadherin-based adhesions. J. Biol. Chem. 279: 30092-30098.
67. Muller, T., Choidas, A., Reichmann, E., and Ullrich, A, 1999, Phosphorylation and free pool of beta-catenin are regulated by tyrosine kinases and tyrosine phosphatases during epithelial cell migration. J. Biol. Chem. 274: 10173-10183.
68. Rosato, R., Veltmaat, J.M., Groffen, J., and Heisterkamp, N., 1998, Involvement of the tyrosine kinase fer in cell adhesion. Molecular & Cellular Biology 18: 5762-5770.
69. Piedra, J., Martinez, D., Castano, J., Miravet, S., Dunach, M., and de Herreros, A.G., 2001, Regulation of beta-catenin structure and activity by tyrosine phosphorylation. J. Biol. Chem. 276: 20436-20443.
70. Allard, P., Zoubeidi, A., Nguyen, L.T., Tessier, S., Tanguay, S., Chevrette, M., Aprikian, A., and Chevalier, S., 2000, Links between Fer tyrosine kinase expression levels and prostate cell proliferation. Molecular & Cellular Endocrinology 159: 63-77.
71. Arregui, C., Pathre, P., Lilien, J., and Balsamo, J., 2000, The nonreceptor tyrosine kinase fer mediates cross-talk between N-cadherin and beta1-integrins. J. Cell Biol. 149: 1263-1274.
72. Krakstad, B.F., Ardawatia, V.V., and Aragay, A.M., 2004, A role for Galpha12/Galpha13 in p120ctn regulation. Proc. Natl. Acad. Sci. 101:10314-9.
73. Kaplan, D.D., Meigs, T.E., and Casey, P.J., 2001, Distinct regions of the cadherin cytoplasmic domain are essential for functional interaction with Galpha 12 and beta-catenin. J. Biol. Chem. 276: 44037-44043.
74. Kurose, H., 2003, Galpha12 and Galpha13 as key regulatory mediator in signal transduction. Life Sci. 74: 155-161.
75. Yan, H.X., He, Y.Q., Dong, H., Zhang, P., Zeng, J.Z., Cao, H.F., Wu, M.C., and Wang, H.Y., 2002, Physical and functional interaction between receptor-like protein tyrosine phosphatase PCP-2 and beta-catenin, Biochemistry 41: 15854-15860.
76. Ukropec, J.A., Hollinger, M.K., Salva, S.M., and Woolkalis, M.J., 2000, SHP2 association with VE-cadherin complexes in human endothelial cells is regulated by thrombin. J. Biol.Chem. 275: 5983-5986.
77. Holsinger, L.J., Ward, K., Duffield, B., Zachwieja, J., and Jallal, B., 2002, The transmembrane receptor protein tyrosine phosphatase DEP1 interacts with p. 120(ctn). Oncogene 21: 7067-7076.
78. Brady-Kalnay, S.M., Mourton, T., Nixon, J.P., Pietz, G.E., Kinch, M., Chen, H., Brackenbury, R., Rimm, D.L., Del Vecchio, R.L., and Tonks, N.K., 1998, Dynamic interaction of PTPmu with multiple cadherins in vivo. J. of Cell Biol. 141: 287-296.
79. Balsamo, J., Leung, T., Ernst, H., Zanin, M.K., and Hoffman, S.X.., 1996, Regulated binding of PTP1B-like phosphatase to N-cadherin: control of cadherin-mediated adhesion by dephosphorylation of beta-catenin. J. Cell Biol. 134: 801-813.
80. Hellberg, C.B., Burden-Gulley, S.M., Pietz, G.E., and Brady-Kalnay, S.M., 2002, Expression of the receptor protein-tyrosine phosphatase, PTPmu, restores E-cadherin-dependent adhesion in human prostate carcinoma cells. J.Biol.Chem. 277: 11165-11173.
81. Chattopadhyay, N., Wang, Z., Ashman, L.K., Brady-Kalnay, S.M., and Kreidberg, J.A., 2003) alpha3beta1 integrin-CD151, a component of the cadherin-catenin complex, regulates PTPmu expression and cell-cell adhesion. J. Cell Biol. 163: 1351-1362.
82. Adams, C.L., Chen, Y.T., Smith, S.J., and Nelson, W.J., 1998, Mechanisms of epithelial cell-cell adhesion and cell compaction revealed by high-resolution tracking of E-cadherin-green fluorescent protein. J. Cell Biol. 142: 1105-1119.

83. Mo, Y.Y., Reynolds, A.B., 1996, Identification of murine p120 isoforms and heterogeneous expression of p120cas isoforms in human tumor cell lines. Cancer Res. 56: 2633-2640.
84. Aono, S., Nakagawa, S., Reynolds, A.B., and Takeichi, M., 1999, p120(ctn) acts as an inhibitory regulator of cadherin function in colon carcinoma cells. J. Cell Biol. 145: 551-562.
85. Berens, M.E., Rief, M.D., Loo, M.A., and Giese, A., 1994, The role of extracellular matrix in human astrocytoma migration and proliferation studied in a microliter scale assay. Clinical & Expt. Metastasis 12: 405-415.
86. Maeda, M., Johnson, K.R., and Wheelock, M.J., 2005, Cadherin switching: essential for behavioral but not morphological changes during an epithelium-to-mesenchyme transition. J.Cell Sci. 118: 873-887.
87. Williams, E.J., Williams, G., Howell, F.V., Skaper, S.D., Walsh, F.S., and Doherty, P., 2001, Identification of an N-cadherin motif that can interact with the fibroblast growth factor receptor and is required for axonal growth. J. Biol. Chem. 276: 43879-43886.
88. Monier-Gavelle, F., Duband, J.L., 1997, Cross talk between adhesion molecules: control of N-cadherin activity by intracellular signals elicited by beta1 and beta3 integrins in migrating neural crest cells. J. Cell Biol. 137: 1663-1681.
89. Arregui, C., Pathre, P., Lilien, J., and Balsamo, J., 2000, The nonreceptor tyrosine kinase fer mediates cross-talk between N-cadherin and beta1-integrins. J. Cell Biol. 149: 1263-1274.
90. Ojakian, G.K., Ratcliffe, D.R., and Schwimmer, R., 2001, Integrin regulation of cell-cell adhesion during epithelial tubule formation. J. Cell Science, 114: 941-952.
91. Frisch, S.M., Ruoslahti, E., 1997, Integrins and anoikis. Current Opinion in Cell Biology 9: 701-706.
92. Tran, N.L., Adams, D.G., Vallincourt, R.L., and Heimark, R.L., 2002, Signaling from N-cadherin increases Bcl-2: regulation of the Phosphatidylinositol 3-Kinase/Akt pathway by homophilic adhesion and actin cytoskeletal organization. J Biol. Chem. 277: 32905-32914.
93. Lambert, M., Choquet, D., and Mege, R.M., 2002, Dynamics of ligand-induced, Rac1-dependent anchoring of cadherins to the actin cytoskeleton. J. Cell Biol. 157: 469-479.
94. Majumder, P.K., Yeh, J.J., George, D.J., Febbo, P.G., Kum, J., Xue, Q., Bikoff, R., Ma, H., Kantoff, P.W., Golub, T.R., Loda, M., and Sellers, W.R.,2003, Prostate intraepithelial neoplasia induced by prostate restricted Akt activation: the MPAKT model. Proc.Natl.Acad.Sci.U.S.A 100: 7841-7846.
95. Kreisberg, J.I., Malik, S.N., Prihoda, T.J., Bedolla, R.G., Troyer, D.A., Kreisberg, S., and Ghosh, P.M., 2004, Phosphorylation of Akt (Ser473) is an excellent predictor of poor clinical outcome in prostate cancer. Cancer Res. 64: 5232-5236.
96. Apakama, I., Robinson, M.C., Walter, N.M., Charlton, R.G., Royds, J.A., Fuller, C.E., Neal, D.E., and Hamdy, F.C., 1996, bcl-2 overexpression combined with p53 protein accumulation correlates with hormone-refractory prostate cancer. British J. Cancer 74: 1258-1262.
97. Colombel, M., Symmans, F., Gil, S., O'Toole, K.M., Chopin, D., Benson, M., Olsson, C.A., Korsmeyer, S., and Buttyan, R., 1993, Detection of the apoptosis-suppressing oncoprotein bc1-2 in hormone-refractory human prostate cancers. American Journal of Pathology 143: 390-400.
98. McDonnell, T.J., Navone, N.M., Troncoso, P., Pisters, L.L., Conti, C, von Eschenbach, A.C., Brisbay, S., and Logothetis, C.J., 1997, Expression of bcl-2 oncoprotein and p53

protein accumulation in bone marrow metastases of androgen independent prostate cancer. J. Urology 157: 569-574.

99. Bruckheimer, E.M., Cho, S., Brisbay, S., Johnson, D.J., Gingrich, J.R., Greenberg, N., and McDonnell, T.J., 2000, The impact of bcl-2 expression and bax deficiency on prostate homeostasis in vivo. Oncogene 19: 2404-2412.

Chapter 4

THE ACTIN CYTOSKELETON AND METASTASIS

Isaac Rabinovitz,[1] and Kaylene J. Simpson[2]
[1]*Department of Pathology, Beth Israel Deaconess Medical Center and Harvard Medical School, Boston, M, USA;* [2]*Department of Cell Biology, Harvard Medical School, Boston, MA, USA*

Abstract: Transformed cells require cell motility to invade adjacent and distant tissues. To move, cells need to operate a dynamic actin cytoskeleton to produce the necessary protrusions and forces that drive the cell forward. Several of the elements of the basic molecular machinery that assemble and operate the actin cytoskeleton have been identified and their function thoroughly characterized. Most of these elements are actin-binding proteins that can be controlled by a network of regulatory molecules that connects the actin cytoskeleton to higher cellular processes. In cancer cells the dynamics and regulation of the actin cytoskeleton may be corrupted at several levels. This review examines several aspects of the actin cytoskeleton that may be affected during transformation and tumor progression.

Key words: actin binding proteins; contractility; cancer; Rho GTPase; cytoskeleton

1. INTRODUCTION

The notion that cancer cells spread by actively migrating into the adjacent stroma, eventually disseminating to distant tissues as metastasis, has been a major motive for interest in exploring the mechanisms of cell movement (1). The general mechanisms of tumor cell migration are not dissimilar to those used by non-neoplastic cells in a wide variety of biological processes such as embryogenesis, immunological response and wound healing (2, 3). To move, cells employ dynamic remodeling of the actin cytoskeleton for the formation of protrusive structures and the generation of forces necessary to produce cell translocation (2). In this

A.E. Cress and R.B. Nagle (eds.), Cell Adhesion and Cytoskeletal Molecules in Metastasis, 69–90.

review we present several aspects of the actin cytoskeleton function and regulation that have an impact in tumor invasion and metastasis.

2. THE BASIC MODEL OF CELL MIGRATION

Directed cell movement was originally described on 2D substrates in the pioneering experiments of Abercrombie (4, 5). The prototype of this kind of migration is the fibroblast which shows a polarized morphology characterized by a fan shaped lamella at the front and an elongated trailing edge at the back. Cell migration is a highly dynamic, cyclical multistep process, (6) requiring a) extension of actin-rich protrusions such as lamellipodia (flat and wide protrusions) or filopodia (thread like protrusions), b) formation of cell adhesive structures near the leading edge that attach and stabilize the protrusion, c) translocation of the cell body forward using the contractive forces generated by the actomyosin system and d) retraction of the tail as a consequence of release of adhesions and active contraction. The initial protrusion is produced by polymerization of the actin cytoskeleton that pushes the membrane forward (7, 8). The protrusion may retract unless stabilized by adhesion to the substrate. This adhesion is usually mediated by integrins, a family of transmembrane proteins that connect the extracellular matrix with the actin cytoskeleton enabling the latter to transmit forces to the substratum, generating traction to pull the cell body forward (9). This type of migration, also known as mesenchymal migration, is not exclusive of fibroblasts and can be seen in epithelial cells when migrating as single cells.

The ability of cells to move in a directed fashion depends mostly on an external source of chemoattractant (chemotaxis) or a substrate gradient (haptotaxis) (10). In the absence of external stimuli the cells usually move in a random fashion, turning frequently, although some cells, such as keratocytes, can move straight for long stretches in a randomly chosen direction as a consequence of their intrinsic ability to maintain lamellar protrusions in that direction (persistence) (11).

3. MECHANISMS OF ACTIN POLYMERIZATION

Lamellipodia and filopodia contain actin filaments generated by polymerization of monomeric actin (G-actin) into double stranded filaments (F-actin). F-actin exists in the lamellipodia as a branched network of fibers, in contrast to the parallel bundles that constitute filopodia. Polymerization of actin in these structures is a dynamic process in which G actin is added onto the faster growing "barbed" end (+) whilst dissociating from the "pointed" end (-), producing a retrograde movement of actin known as treadmilling that is ATP-dependent (8, 12, 13). The elongation of the protrusion results from an imbalance in the rates of actin polymerization and depolymerization, favoring the former. This balance is highly regulated depending on the specific requirement of the cell. In resting cells there is little growth of actin filaments, the barbed ends are blocked by capping proteins (gelsolin and capping protein) and the pool of monomeric actin is prevented from polymerizing by sequestering proteins (profilin, thymosin β4) (14, 15). Upon external stimulation, the existing actin filaments get uncapped and severed, generating new nucleation sites containing free barbed ends to which monomeric actin can be added.

Three nucleation mechanisms have been described which relate to the type of actin arrangement they produce. These nucleation processes depend on the activity of a variety of proteins, some of which are functionally and structurally related to actin. Branched networks of F-actin produced at the leading edge of lamellipodia depend on the concerted action of the Arp2/3 complex and WASP family members (16). The Arp2/3 complex contains seven subunits, of which Arp2 and Arp3 are related to actin (17). This complex generates a Y-shaped junction on uncapped filaments resulting in a branched network (as opposed to filopodia, in which no branching occurs). The network is stabilized by cortactin (18, 19).

Arp2/3 is highly regulated and is activated by uncapped F-actin filaments, ATP and proteins of the WASP family. Chemoattractant generated signals activate Arp2/3 through the WASP family (20) of which five members have been identified; WASP itself (Wiscott Aldrich syndrome protein), N-WASP and WAVE1, 2 and 3 (20, 21). These proteins respond to signals elicited through the Rho GTPases Cdc42 and Rac1. Cdc42 is directly recruited by WASP and N-WASP, while Rac1 conveys its message to WAVE through Nck and JSPC300 (22). The WASP family has additional domains that bind regulatory phosphatidylinositol 4,5 biphosphate thereby localizing the Arp2/3/WASP complex to the membrane, and profilin, which supplies the monomeric actin for polymerization (20).

A second group of proteins involved in actin nucleation is the Ena/VASP family that includes Ena (Mena), VASP and EVL (Ena-VASP-like) (23). These proteins are primarily positioned in lamellipodia and, unlike Arp2/3, also at the tips of filopodia, although they can be found in focal adhesions and adherens junctions. The Ena/VASP family can interact with profilin and actin and have been shown to increase nucleation of actin *in vitro*. The mechanism of action of these nucleating proteins is less understood. Interestingly, fibroblasts that lack Ena/VASP move straight longer distances (persistence). In contrast, cells that have Ena/VASP directed to the plasma membrane exhibit an increase in both the rate of protrusion and retraction of lamellipodia, resulting in a net decrease in translocation (24, 25). These observations have led to the idea that Ena/VASP proteins enhance actin polymerization at the membrane by acting as anti-capping proteins. Growth factor signals find their way to Ena/VASP proteins through cAMP-dependent protein kinase A (PKA), which phosphorylates and inhibits their actin nucleation activity. Recently, LPD (lamellipodin) was identified as an Ena/VASP associated protein necessary for lamellipodial protrusion (26).

A third group is the Diaphanous-related formin homology proteins: mDia1, 2 and 3, which are involved in the control of stress fiber and focal adhesion formation downstream of Rho and Rho Kinase (ROCK) (27, 28). mDia proteins nucleate unbranched actin filaments *in vitro* and bind to profilin. Rho GTPase binds to mDia proteins breaking intramolecular interactions that maintain mDia inactive (29).

Polymerization of actin occurs only if the growing ends are uncapped. Gelsolin is one of the capping proteins that normally prevents actin polymerization in resting cells (15, 30). A rise in Ca2+ activates gelsolin, promoting binding to actin, severing of filaments and capping. A subsequent increase in polyphosphoinositides detaches gelsolin from the actin filaments, uncapping them and producing new nucleation sites.

While the forementioned proteins regulate polymerization at the growing (+) end of the actin filaments the ADF/cofilin family regulates the rate of actin depolymerization at the pointed (-) end by enhancing the rate of dissociation of ADP-actin at these ends (14, 31). Although this activity would reduce the number and size of actin filaments, ADF/cofilin has a weak severing activity, resulting in the formation of new nucleation sites and therefore an increase in actin polymerization. ADF/cofilin is regulated by phosphorylation and competitive phosphoinositide binding. LIM-kinases phosphorylate and inactivate ADF/cofilin (31) through growth factor induced regulation of Rho GTPases. Recently a phosphatase, chronophin, has been identified as a regulator of ADF/cofilin (32). Chronophin directly dephosphorylates ADF/cofilin and its absence results in the stabilization of stress fibers as well as massive cell division defects.

4. SIGNALING PATHWAYS REGULATING ACTIN POLYMERIZATION AND CONTRACTILITY

Physiological and pathological processes where cell migration is involved need to modulate the function and organization of the actin cytoskeleton in a timely and coordinated manner (2, 6). Crucial in our understanding of the regulation of the actin cytoskeleton was the discovery of the Rho-family of GTPases (33, 34). These proteins behave as molecular switches cycling between GTP and GDP bound forms in response to stimuli such as growth factors that induce migration. Rho GTPases are activated by exchange of GDP for GTP via guanine nucleotide exchange factors (GEFs), enabling interactions with specific downstream effectors that modify the actin cytoskeleton function and organization. They are inactivated through the action of guanine activating proteins (GAPs). The three original members of this family, RhoA, Rac1 and Cdc42, where found to be critical regulators of stress fibers, lamellipodia and filopodia respectively (33). As mentioned above, major targets for Rac1 and Cdc42 are the WASP and WAVE family of Arp2/3 complex activators (20, 21). Rac1 stimulates lamellipodia protrusion by activating WAVE proteins, while Cdc42 binds to WASP and together they activate Arp2/3. WAVE and WASPS may themselves regulate the activity of Rac and Cdc42 by binding to GAPs and GEFs, creating feedback loops that regulate actin polymerization.

Establishing cell polarity is important to achieve efficient migration (2). Rho GTPases, phosphoinositide 3-kinases, integrin microtubules and vesicular transport play an important role in establishing polarization (35). In addition to promoting actin polymerization, Cdc42 is crucial in determining and maintaining polarization, with modification of its expression disrupting polarization (36, 37). One of the mechanisms used by Cdc42 to generate polarity is to limit the sites of protrusion. This GTPase can also modulate the polarity by redistributing the microtubule-organizing center (MTOC) in front of the nucleus facing the leading edge (38). This orientation of the MTOC helps microtubules penetrate the lamella, stimulating further protrusion in that direction and increasing persistence (39). Cdc42 may also work together with PI3K and PTEN to maintain polarity. PI3K phosphoinositide products accumulate at the leading edge of cells exposed to chemoattractants (40, 41) and are necessary for Cdc42 to localize to the leading edge (42). PTEN functions to counteract PI3K by dephosphorylating PI3K products. Interestingly, Cdc42 is thought to be involved in the exclusion of PTEN from the leading edge, restricting it to the sides and the trailing edge (42). Thus Cdc42 and PI3K generate a positive loop that promotes accumulation of phosphoinositides at the leading edge. This pathway also leads to increased actin polymerization through activation of RacGEFs by phosphoinositides (43). This activates Rac at the leading edge, which in addition to its interaction with Ena/VASP proteins that promote actin polymerization, it establishes a positive polarization feedback loop by reinforcing the activity of PI3K, stabilizing microtubules, promoting recruitment of integrins and forming new adhesions (44, 45).

RhoA and myosin-light chain kinase (MLCK) are the major regulators of actin cytoskeleton contractility, through the direct or indirect phosphorylation of the myosin light chain, activating myosin and generating contractility. The contractility induced by RhoA is necessary for the production of stress fibers and focal adhesions (46, 47). Several downstream effectors of RhoA have been described, including ROCK and mDia1. ROCK stimulates myosin II–driven contractility through phosphorylation and inactivation of the myosin light chain phosphatase (48, 49) and by direct phosphorylation of the myosin light chain (MLC) (50). Inhibition of ROCK function by chemical inhibitors or dominant negative mutants prevents the formation of focal contacts (51, 52), but not of focal complexes. After lamellipodia protrude, the initial adhesion (focal complex) is dependent on Rac1, but maturation into a focal adhesion depends on RhoA and contractility. The maturation of focal adhesions can be rendered independent of ROCK if external forces are applied, in which case mDia1 is necessary and sufficient to produce the maturation of the focal adhesion (53). RhoA induced contractility during cell migration is mostly restricted to the trailing edge as Cdc42 and Rac1 at the leading edge decrease RhoA activity (54). RhoA activation at the rear of the cell results in the generation of tension on the rear adhesions and helps detachment of this region. Inhibition of RhoA results in the formation of elongated tails that do not detach, reducing net migration (55).

5. CELL MOTILITY IN TUMOR INVASION AND METASTASIS

Historically, evidence for tumor cell movement was initially inferred from the analysis of cell positions in tissue sections obtained from histological specimens (56, 57). The position of single cancer cells at some distance from the invasion front was used as the main argument for locomotion. The problem with this static morphology approach was that the possibility of passive shifting could not be ruled out. For example, detached tumor cells could be transported passively by the streaming forces generated by the higher interstitial pressure in the tumor as compared to the normal surrounding tissue (57). Complicating the picture, a great number of histological studies using serial sectioning to reconstruct the architecture of the whole tumor, demonstrated that in most cases of human carcinoma, a cohesive structure was the most common form of invasion, while single cells were rarely seen and only at very late stages of the tumor. These type of studies suggested that in human carcinomas, at least in the initial stages of invasion, migration of collective cells thrusting out wedges, tongues or sheets would be the prevailing form of migration. This type of movement would resemble the epibolic morphogenetic movements of surface cells seen in the amphibian egg (58). Again, these studies could not rule out the possibility that the collective movement of carcinoma cells was a consequence of passive displacement, for example, the passive growth of a tumor extending its mass into an anatomic path of least resistance.

Microcinematography provided direct evidence of carcinoma cell movement using an *in vivo* experimental system. The studies pioneered by Wood showed that carcinoma cells injected directly into the rabbit ear vasculature could actively move out of the vessels (59). Time lapse filming was also used by others to demonstrate that the metastatic potential of carcinoma cells correlates with their ability to extravasate in this type of experiments, although this was not always the case (58).

The use of digital imaging, new molecular biology techniques and improved model systems has allowed investigators to examine more closely the role of cell movement during the metastatic cascade. An example is the analysis of intravasation, a step in the metastatic cascade in which primary tumor cells enter blood vessels. Using confocal time lapse microscopy of GFP labeled cells Segall et al. were able to study the motile characteristics of mammary carcinoma cells with different intravasation potential (60, 61). Interestingly, both intravasating and non-intravasating cells showed similar motile characteristics, namely equal protrusive activity, however, the metastatic cells oriented better towards blood vessels, indicating that motility *per se* is not enough to produce metastasis and that chemotactic factors, such as growth factors secreted by endothelial cells, may be needed to maximize intravasation.

The morphology of a variety of tumor cells migrating *in vivo* or in 3D matrices *in vitro* is substantially different from that observed in 2D cultures. The cells are more rounded, the protrusions are pseudopodial rather than lamellar, the adhesive structures such as focal adhesions are reduced and stress fibers are absent (62). This has led to the idea that migration of some tumor cells may resemble the ameboid movement of leukocytes rather than mesenchymal cells (63). One of the most important differences between the ameboid and mesenchymal types of migration is the way the cells generate the anchorage necessary for traction. In the case of cells with a mesenchymal type of movement the traction is transmitted through adhesive structures anchored to the substrate (62). In contrast, cells embedded within a 3D substrate showing ameboid type of movement gain non-adhesive anchorage or “mechanical anchorage” by pushing narrow protrusions through gaps in the gel meshwork and expanding the protrusion so that it cannot be easily withdrawn, therefore gaining leverage for traction (62). For cells that can move quickly using ameboid movement, such as neutrophils, forming adhesions slows their migration. This type of migration has been observed in several experimental tumors, such as V2 kidney carcinoma and Ras transformed mammary carcinoma (59, 60). Ameboid movement has also been observed in lymphoma and leukemia cells (64). Some static morphology studies of human carcinoma suggest that ameboid movement may occur during invasion. For example, tumor cells caught "in fragranti" invading blood vessels have morphologies consistent with ameboid movement (56). Future studies are needed to understand better this type of movement in carcinomas.

Collective migration of cells is well documented in several stages of embryonic morphogenesis and during wound healing (58). This type of migration has also been shown in groups of tumor cells grown *in vitro* (65, 66). In these studies the cells at the periphery of the group generate traction through lamellipodial or pseudopodial activity, with the cells behind them being dragged passively. In 3D matrices, these experimental tumors may resemble the tongues of invasion observed in a wide variety of human carcinoma and even provide a mechanism for the formation of isolated clusters of cells detached from the main mass of the tumor. However, no direct observation of collective movement has been possible in human tumors and more studies are needed to show that collective invasion is not a consequence of a group of cells growing passively into paths of least resistance. Importantly, the experimental 3D models describing collective invasion *in vitro* may not reflect the reality of well differentiated invasive tumors which usually have a well preserved basement membrane (67) that may hinder the protrusive activity seen in experimental models.

6. DEREGULATION OF ACTIN POLYMERIZATION AND CONTRACTILITY DURING INVASION AND METASTASIS

Considering the critical role of cell migration, and hence the actin cytoskeleton in invasion and metastasis it is not surprising that a substantial number of alterations in the function of the actin cytoskeleton have been described. These changes can be observed at different levels and range from a dysfunction in the cytoskeleton basic building blocks, the assembling machinery, and higher level regulators.

6a. Alterations in the basic assembling machinery of the actin cytoskeleton in cancer

β-actin. A number of studies report mutations in the basic unit of the cytoskeleton (68, 69). A mutation in G244D is thought to enhance the tumorigenic capability of immortalized human fibroblasts inoculated in rodent models. In melanoma cells the mutation R28L has been associated with tumor progression in mice.

Myosin II. No mutations have been described for the basic motor of the actin cytoskeleton. Yet, it is an important target of regulatory proteins involved in tumor progression.

Arp2/3. There are only a few studies of Arp2/3 in cancer. A reduction in the expression of Arp2/3 has been observed in gastric tumors (70). In this study, 31 primary cancer samples showed decreased expression of at least one subunit, and 25 samples showed decreased expressions of four or more of the seven subunits. In contrast, immunohisotochemical analysis of colorectal tumors showed that both carcinoma and associated stromal cells had elevated Arp2/3 expression with a higher degree of atypia (71). More studies are needed to clarify the role of Arp2/3 in cancer.

WASP/WAVE. Defects in these proteins severely affect the immune system as observed in early studies of the Wiskott Aldrich Syndrome, which results from mutations in the WAS gene and is characterized by eczema, thrombocytopenia and immunodeficiency. There are several studies suggesting the involvement of the WASP/WAVE family in cancer, although a primary defect in the protein has not been reported. For example, in highly invasive MDA-MB-231 breast carcinoma cells WAVE3 knockdown results in the inhibition of cell motility and invasion, coupled with increased actin stress fiber formation, as well as reorganization of focal adhesion complexes. Knockdown of WAVE3 also affects the expression of phospho-p38 MAPK and metalloproteinases (72). In a different study malignant B16F10 mouse melanoma cells, which are highly metastatic, expressed more WAVE1 and WAVE2 proteins and showed higher Rac activity than B16 parental cells, which are neither invasive nor metastatic. Moreover, membrane ruffling, cell motility, invasion and metastasis of the B16F10 cells were suppressed by WAVE2 RNA interference (RNAi) (73). To define mechanisms by which WASP/WAVE proteins promote invasion, the sites of N-WASP activity during cell motility and invasion in carcinoma cells were examined using a fluorescence resonance energy transfer (FRET) biosensor that distinguishes between the active and inactive conformations of N-WASP. This study showed N-WASP is involved in lamellipodia extension, where it is activated at the leading edge, as well as in invadopodia formation where it is activated at the base. Invadopodia are membrane protrusions that extend deeply into the ECM promoting degradation (74, 75). The branching and architecture of tumors may also be affected by WASP/WAVE proteins. Madin-Darby canine kidney (MDCK) epithelial cells form branching tubules and are invasive when cultured with hepatocyte growth factor (HGF) in collagen gels. A dominant-negative form of N-WASP inhibited the formation of branching tubules and invasion in response to HGF (76).

Gelsolin. Gelsolin is a widely distributed actin binding protein involved in controlling cell morphology, motility, signaling and apoptosis (15, 30). Its role in cancer is still inconclusive. A reduction in gelsolin expression has been observed in diverse types of tumors, with most of these studies showing an inverse correlation with malignancy, suggesting it may behave as a tumor suppressor (77-80). Moreover, gene therapy that restores gelsolin expression in bladder carcinoma cells inoculated in nude mice can notably reduce tumorigenesis (81). In contrast with these studies, increased gelsolin expression has been detected in breast cancer (82). Supporting the idea that gelsolin is a tumor promoter rather than a suppressor, is the fact that the expression of gelsolin in MDCK cells promotes Ras/Rac-dependent invasion into collagen type I and chick heart fragments (83). Clearly more studies are needed to clarify the role of gelsolin in cancer.

ADF/Cofilin. This protein may play an important role in cancer at multiple levels. As mentioned, the ADF/Cofilin family of actin-binding proteins increase microfilament dynamics by a filament-severing activity and by increasing the rate at which actin monomers leave the pointed (-) end of the filament, facilitating cell movement (31). The involvement of ADF/cofilin in cancer was initially suggested by the finding that in adenocarcinoma cells it was required to produce lamellipodia (84). Other studies have supported this idea, with overexpression of ADF/cofilin correlating with increased cell migration in glioblastoma cells (85). The position of ADF/cofilin within the cell may be critical for its involvement in cancer. In this regard, ADF/cofilin has been shown to be present in invadopodia and be important for invadopodia maturation (75). Evidence for direct deregulation of ADF/cofilin in human cancer is still lacking, although increased levels have been found in ovarian tumors by cDNA-array analysis (86). More likely, ADF/cofilin is a target of signaling pathways that promote invasion. For example, ADF/cofilin has been shown to participate in the reorganization of the cytoskeleton that occurs in Ras transformed cells. In Ras transformed cells, ADF/cofilin phosphorylation is compromised by inhibitory action of p21(Cip1) on the ROCK/LIM/cofilin pathway (87). ADF/Cofilin is inactivated by serine phosphorylation by LIM kinases, which lie downstream of the Rho family GTPases being activated by phosphorylation by Rho kinase PAK (14).

Cortactin. Cortactin is an important molecular scaffold for actin assembly and organization. It is an F-actin binding protein that activates Arp2/3 complex and is localized within lamellipodia (18, 19). Cortactin-knockdown cells have a selective defect in the persistence of lamellipodial protrusions (19). It binds directly to Arp2/3 and can synergize with WASP family proteins in the stimulation of actin polymerization. Cortactin is recruited by the Arp2/3 complex to lamellipodia and binds with a higher affinity to ATP F-actin than to ADP-F-actin (19). It also stabilizes Arp2/3 networks by inhibiting debranching. Cortactin is probably also an integrator of signaling pathways that regulate actin polymerization as it is a substrate for Src and other protein tyrosine kinases involved in cell motility, where its phosphorylation on tyrosines is required for cell movement and metastasis. The involvement of cortactin in cancer was suspected initially by the fact that gene amplification of chromosome 11q13 in breast cancer and squamous carcinomas of the head and neck results in frequent overexpression of cortactin (88, 89). In experimental systems, cortactin overexpressing cells have been shown more motile and invasive. Overexpression of cortactin in a non-metastatic HCC cell line increased cell motility, and resulted in metastasis in an orthotopic model (90). Cortactin has been shown to be important in the formation of invadopodia. Anti-cortactin antibodies block matrix degradation at invadopodia (91). In addition it is present in podosomes, which are membrane invaginations surrounded by an actin network that also contains cortactin (92). Cortactin is also involved in coupling the endocytic machinery to dynamic actin networks, and it has been shown that overexpression of cortactin may inhibit the down-regulation of growth factor receptors such as EGFR which may impact further reorganization of the actin cytoskeleton (93).

MIM. This protein was originally described as a protein whose mRNA was Missing in Metastasis (MIM), as it was absent in metastatic bladder carcinoma cell lines (94). The MIM gene encodes an actin binding protein that is expressed at low levels in a subset of malignant cell lines. It colocalizes and interacts directly with cortactin (95) and promotes cortactin and Arp2/3 complex-mediated actin polymerization. Full-length MIM binds to G-actin and inhibits N-WASP actin polymerization. Overexpression of MIM inhibited the motility of NIH3T3 fibroblasts resulting in the disappearance of actin stress fibers and appearance of abnormal actin filament structures(95). The motility was restored in these cells with N-WASP. However, a MIM mutant unable to bind G-actin, enhanced cell motility. In contrast, preventing MIM binding to cortactin, increases MIM-mediated inhibition of cell motility. (95). A variant MIM-B induces actin-rich protrusions and promotes disassembly of actin stress fibers. MIM-B is an actin-binding protein, probably via a WASP-homology 2 domain (actin monomer-binding motif) and interacts with the cytoplasmic domain of protein tyrosine phosphatase (PTP)δ (96). Thus, MIM-B may be a regulator of actin assembly downstream of tyrosine kinase signalling and this activity may explain the involvement of MIM in the metastasis of cancer cells. (96). Recombinant MIM interacts with actin monomers and inhibits actin filament nucleation *in vitro*. However, the MIM/ATP-G-actin complex can participate in actin filament assembly at the barbed end (97). It will be interesting to define what functions of this tumor suppressor are directly related to the invasive phenotype.

6b. The regulators of the actomyosin system in cancer

Signals generated by growth factors, cytokines, cell adhesion receptors and other surface receptors converge onto the Rho GTPase family of proteins that in turn regulate actin cytoskeleton polymerization and contractility.

Several members of this family are thought to participate in human cancer not only at the level of cytoskeletal organization, but also at the levels of gene expression, cell proliferation and survival (98-100). To date, no mutations have been detected in the Rho GTPase members, however increased activity or expression is commonly observed in several types of tumors, including breast, colon, pancreas, and squamous cell carcinomas, as well as melanomas, correlating with increased malignancy. There are eleven Rho specific isoforms, and whilst RhoA has been the most characterized isoform, recent attention has been given to the highly homologous RhoB and RhoC isoforms. It is now clear that all Rho proteins are not equal and these proteins have been shown to have distinct roles in both cytoskeletal dynamics and caner. In inflammatory breast carcinoma (101) and melanoma (102) cells, RhoC is overexpressed, correlating with the metastatic potential of the cells. Moreover, genetic manipulation of weakly metastatic cells to overexpress RhoC increases their metastatic potential (102, 103). These studies have been supported in RhoC-deficient mice whereby tumor development remains unaffected and motility as well as metastasis were inhibited (104), and by RNAi in invasive breast carcinoma cells (105). Interestingly, RhoC has also been implicated in regulation of tumor angiogenesis (106) and RhoB has been shown to play a developmental role in endothelial cell survival during vasculature development (107).

Inhibition of RhoA, Rac1 or Cdc42 through dominant-negative approaches can impede transformation of fibroblasts by Ras (98). While dominant-negative and constitutively active approaches together with bacterial toxin treatments and biochemical inhibitors have been conventional tools to study Rho functionality, they cannot distinguish between isoforms due to high sequence similarity in the functional regions of the genes. RNAi has now made this possible. Knockdown of RhoA and RhoC in invasive breast carcinoma cells revealed independent and co-dependent functions for these genes, with increased motility observed after knockdown of RhoA, which was attributed to increased RhoC activity (105).

Inhibition of Rho effectors can also efficiently reduce carcinoma cell migration. For example, ROCK, which induces myosin contraction through direct and indirect phosphorylation of the myosin light chain, can be inhibited using the pharmacological inhibitor Y27632 resulting in reduced migration of breast and prostate carcinoma cells (108, 109).

In several types of tumors the proteins that regulate the GTP/GDP cycle of Rho GTPases may function inadequately. For example, increase in the activity of GEFs such as Tiam1, βPIX and Vav1 can induce tumors and have been isolated in screens for transforming genes (99). Tiam1 is a Rac-specific GEF and has been shown to be mutated in some renal carcinomas, and can inhibit invasion of renal carcinoma cells *in vitro* (110, 111). GAPs such as p190RhoGAP can act as tumor suppressors. For example, p190 RhoGAP is activated by Src resulting in the inhibition of Rho, acting as a tumor suppressor in gliomas (112, 113).

An increase in Rho activity may be a consequence of upstream dysregulation. An important target of growth factors and cytokines is PI3K, whose products such as PtdIns(3,4,5)P3 can mediate the activation of Rho GTPases and direct cell motility (114). Integrins can differentially activate RhoA or Rac1 in carcinoma cells. For example, in a human squamous carcinoma model, the $\alpha 3\beta 1$ integrin may inhibit RhoA and stimulate Rac1 when cells attach to laminin resulting in increased migration, while the $\alpha 2\beta 1$ integrin may stimulate RhoA when cells attach to collagen and reduce migration (115), highlighting the importance of the tumor environment to determine the activity or Rho GTPases.

RhoA is critical in the regulation of forces generated by the cytoskeleton and transmitted to the substrate by integrins. These forces have profound effects in developmental processes such as embryonic branching, determining cell behavior and architecture. Tissue compliance is important in determining these forces and can alter morphogenesis. Malignant transformation may be associated with changes in the tissue tension and ECM stiffening, probably explaining the increase in RhoA expression observed in certain tumors such as breast (116). The RhoA dependent generation of force can impact the reorganization of basement membranes, the integrity of which is altered during invasion. Several tumor cells show increased Rho-dependent ability to reorganize the basement membrane, which could potentially contribute to the dissemination of the cells (117, 118). The regulation of RhoA by integrins can also affect the persistence in cell migration. In a recent study, $\alpha v\beta 3$ integrins that mediate attachment to fibronectin promote a persistent form of migration, which can be changed to a random type of migration when RhoA is stimulated by the integrin $\alpha 5\beta 1$, resulting in the inhibition of cofilin (119).

Inhibition of Rac1 function or expression by using dominant negative or RNAi strategies results in inhibition of cell migration and invasive behavior in some cell types, such as breast carcinoma and glioma cells (120, 121). Although the constitutively activated form does not necessarily increase migration, as is the case for the MDA-MB-435 cells (122), in some cases it can inhibit migration, as seen in HeLa cervical carcinoma cells or clear Ca-28 renal carcinoma cells (111, 123). A possible explanation for this discrepancy is that Rac may need to actively cycle between the GTP and GDP bound forms in order to be functional. In melanoma cells, constitutively active Rac1 can induce invasion, and WAVE2 was identified as the primary downstream effector mediating this response (73). The collaboration of the different Rho GTPases can be observed in several instances, for example, Cdc42 can collaborate with Rho through MRCK (myotonic dystrophy kinase-related Cdc42-binding kinase) signalling to inhibit the myosin light chain phosphatase, increasing the phosphorylation of MLC resulting in increasing contractility and invasive ability (124).

7. CONCLUSIONS AND PERSPECTIVE

Considerable advances have contributed to our understanding of how the actin cytoskeleton works and is regulated. Research on the actin cytoskeleton of the past few years has provided important and exciting clues on the mechanisms of cell migration and carcinoma invasion. The discovery of Arp2/3, WASP and Ena/VASP offer reliable explanations about the fine working assembly machinery of the actin cytoskeleton. The studies on the Rho GTPase family have provided a clear picture of the regulatory network that controls the actin cytoskeleton and how signals of different hierarchy converge to control the function of the actomyosin system. Several of these proteins are affected during tumor progression and their effect is not only seen in cell migration and invasion but also in other cell functions such as proliferation, apoptosis, differentiation and gene expression. Some of the proteins involved in the assembly or regulation of the actin cytoskeleton could be potential therapeutic targets. The use of *in vivo* models and mouse genetics should be useful to determine interactions between the different elements that integrate the actomyosin system. A challenge for the future is to determine how genes involved in tumor progression may disturb the actin cytoskeleton to induce an invasive phenotype in tumor cells. This will greatly aid the design of pharmacologic or genetic agents that may target the function of the actin cytoskeleton in a rational way to prevent cell dissemination.

ACKNOWLEDGEMENTS

Funding for the authors' work described in this review was supported by NIH grants CA88919 (IR) and DOD W81XWH-04-1-0360 (KJS).

REFERENCES

1. Stetler-Stevenson, W.G., Aznavoorian, S., and Liotta, L.A. Tumor cell interactions with the extracellular matrix during invasion and metastasis. Annual Review of Cell Biology, 9: 541-573, 1993.
2. Ridley, A.J., Schwartz, M.A., Burridge, K., Firtel, R.A., Ginsberg, M.H., Borisy, G., Parsons, J.T., and Horwitz, A.R. Cell migration: integrating signals from front to back. Science, 302: 1704-1709, 2003.
3. Yamaguchi, H., Wyckoff, J., and Condeelis, J. Cell migration in tumors. Curr Opin Cell Biol, 17: 559-564, 2005.
4. Abercrombie, M., Heaysman, J.E., and Pegrum, S.M. The locomotion of fibroblasts in culture. I. Movements of the leading edge. Exp Cell Res, 59: 393-398, 1970.
5. Abercrombie, M., Heaysman, J.E., and Pegrum, S.M. The locomotion of fibroblasts in culture. II. "Ruffling". Exp Cell Res, 60: 437-444, 1970.
6. Lauffenburger, D.A. and Horwitz, A.F. Cell migration - a physically integrated molecular process. Cell, 84: 359-369, 1996.
7. Borisy, G.G. and Svitkina, T.M. Actin machinery: pushing the envelope. Curr Opin Cell Biol, 12: 104-112, 2000.
8. Pollard, T.D. and Borisy, G.G. Cellular motility driven by assembly and disassembly of actin filaments. Cell, 112: 453-465, 2003.
9. Hynes, R. O. Integrins: versatility, modulation, and signaling in cell adhesion. Cell, 69: 11-25, 1992.
10. Harms, B.D., Bassi, G.M., Horwitz, A.R., and Lauffenburger, D.A. Directional persistence of EGF-induced cell migration is associated with stabilization of lamellipodial protrusions. Biophys J, 88: 1479-1488, 2005.
11. Verkhovsky, A.B., Svitkina, T.M., and Borisy, G.G. Self-polarization and directional motility of cytoplasm. Curr Biol, 9: 11-20, 1999.
12. Wang, Y.L. Exchange of actin subunits at the leading edge of living fibroblasts: possible role of treadmilling. J Cell Biol, 101: 597-602, 1985.
13. Pollard, T.D., Blanchoin, L., and Mullins, R.D. Molecular mechanisms controlling actin filament dynamics in nonmuscle cells. Annu Rev Biophys Biomol Struct, 29: 545-576, 2000.

14. Winder, S.J. and Ayscough, K.R. Actin-binding proteins. J Cell Sci, 118: 651-654, 2005.
15. dos Remedios, C.G., Chhabra, D., Kekic, M., Dedova, I.V., Tsubakihara, M., Berry, D.A., and Nosworthy, N.J. Actin binding proteins: regulation of cytoskeletal microfilaments. Physiol Rev, 83: 433-473, 2003.
16. Pollard, T.D. and Beltzner, C.C. Structure and function of the Arp2/3 complex. Curr Opin Struct Biol, 12: 768-774, 2002.
17. Machesky, L.M. and Gould, K.L. The Arp2/3 complex: a multifunctional actin organizer. Curr Opin Cell Biol, 11: 117-121, 1999.
18. Weed, S.A. and Parsons, J.T. Cortactin: coupling membrane dynamics to cortical actin assembly. Oncogene, 20: 6418-6434, 2001.
19. Bryce, N.S., Clark, E.S., Leysath, J.L., Currie, J.D., Webb, D.J., and Weaver, A.M. Cortactin promotes cell motility by enhancing lamellipodial persistence. Curr Biol, 15: 1276-1285, 2005.
20. Stradal, T.E., Rottner, K., Disanza, A., Confalonieri, S., Innocenti, M., and Scita, G. Regulation of actin dynamics by WASP and WAVE family proteins. Trends Cell Biol, 14: 303-311, 2004.
21. Takenawa, T. and Miki, H. WASP and WAVE family proteins: key molecules for rapid rearrangement of cortical actin filaments and cell movement. J Cell Sci, 114: 1801-1809, 2001.
22. Eden, S., Rohatgi, R., Podtelejnikov, A.V., Mann, M., and Kirschner, M.W. Mechanism of regulation of WAVE1-induced actin nucleation by Rac1 and Nck. Nature, 418: 790-793, 2002.
23. Krause, M., Dent, E.W., Bear, J.E., Loureiro, J.J., and Gertler, F.B. Ena/VASP proteins: regulators of the actin cytoskeleton and cell migration. Annu Rev Cell Dev Biol, 19: 541-564, 2003.
24. Bear, J.E., Loureiro, J.J., Libova, I., Fassler, R., Wehland, J., and Gertler, F.B. Negative regulation of fibroblast motility by Ena/VASP proteins. Cell, 101: 717-728, 2000.
25. Bear, J.E., Svitkina, T.M., Krause, M., Schafer, D.A., Loureiro, J.J., Strasser, G.A., Maly, I.V., Chaga, O.Y., Cooper, J.A., Borisy, G.G., and Gertler, F.B. Antagonism between Ena/VASP proteins and actin filament capping regulates fibroblast motility. Cell, 109: 509-521, 2002.
26. Krause, M., Leslie, J.D., Stewart, M., Lafuente, E.M., Valderrama, F., Jagannathan, R., Strasser, G.A., Rubinson, D.A., Liu, H., Way, M., Yaffe, M.B., Boussiotis, V.A., and Gertler, F.B. Lamellipodin, an Ena/VASP ligand, is implicated in the regulation of lamellipodial dynamics. Dev Cell, 7: 571-583, 2004.
27. Alberts, A.S. Diaphanous-related Formin homology proteins. Curr Biol, 12: R796, 2002.
28. Watanabe, N. and Higashida, C. Formins: processive cappers of growing actin filaments. Exp Cell Res, 301: 16-22, 2004.
29. Alberts, A.S. Identification of a carboxyl-terminal diaphanous-related formin homology protein autoregulatory domain. J Biol Chem, 276: 2824-2830, 2001.
30. Silacci, P., Mazzolai, L., Gauci, C., Stergiopulos, N., Yin, H.L., and Hayoz, D. Gelsolin superfamily proteins: key regulators of cellular functions. Cell Mol Life Sci, 61: 2614-2623, 2004.
31. Bamburg, J.R. and Wiggan, O.P. ADF/cofilin and actin dynamics in disease. Trends Cell Biol, 12: 598-605, 2002.
32. Gohla, A., Birkenfeld, J., and Bokoch, G.M. Chronophin, a novel HAD-type serine protein phosphatase, regulates cofilin-dependent actin dynamics. Nat Cell Biol, 7: 21-29, 2005.

33. Hall, A. Rho GTPases and the actin cytoskeleton. Science, 279: 509-514, 1998.
34. Jaffe, A.B. and Hall, A. RHO GTPASES: Biochemistry and Biology. Annu Rev Cell Dev Biol, 21: 247-269, 2005.
35. Fukata, M., Nakagawa, M., and Kaibuchi, K. Roles of Rho-family GTPases in cell polarisation and directional migration. Curr Opin Cell Biol, 15: 590-597, 2003.
36. Etienne-Manneville, S. and Hall, A. Cdc42 regulates GSK-3beta and adenomatous polyposis coli to control cell polarity. Nature, 421: 753-756, 2003.
37. Etienne-Manneville, S. and Hall, A. Rho GTPases in cell biology. Nature, 420: 629-635, 2002.
38. Lee, J.S., Chang, M.I., Tseng, Y., and Wirtz, D. Cdc42 mediates nucleus movement and MTOC polarization in Swiss 3T3 fibroblasts under mechanical shear stress. Mol Biol Cell, 16: 871-880, 2005.
39. Rodriguez, O.C., Schaefer, A.W., Mandato, C.A., Forscher, P., Bement, W.M., and Waterman-Storer, C.M. Conserved microtubule-actin interactions in cell movement and morphogenesis. Nat Cell Biol, 5: 599-609, 2003.
40. Merlot, S. and Firtel, R.A. Leading the way: Directional sensing through phosphatidylinositol 3-kinase and other signaling pathways. J Cell Sci, 116: 3471-3478, 2003.
41. Devreotes, P. and Janetopoulos, C. Eukaryotic chemotaxis: distinctions between directional sensing and polarization. J Biol Chem, 278: 20445-20448, 2003.
42. Li, Z., Hannigan, M., Mo, Z., Liu, B., Lu, W., Wu, Y., Smrcka, A.V., Wu, G., Li, L., Liu, M., Huang, C.K., and Wu, D. Directional sensing requires G beta gamma-mediated PAK1 and PIX alpha-dependent activation of Cdc42. Cell, 114: 215-227, 2003.
43. Welch, H.C., Coadwell, W.J., Stephens, L.R., and Hawkins, P.T. Phosphoinositide 3-kinase-dependent activation of Rac. FEBS Lett, 546: 93-97, 2003.
44. Kiosses, W.B., Shattil, S.J., Pampori, N., and Schwartz, M.A. Rac recruits high-affinity integrin alphavbeta3 to lamellipodia in endothelial cell migration. Nat Cell Biol, 3: 316-320, 2001.
45. Schwartz, M. Rho signalling at a glance. J Cell Sci, 117: 5457-5458, 2004.
46. Burridge, K. and Chrzanowska-Wodnicka, M. Focal adhesions, contractility, and signaling. Annu Rev Cell Dev Biol, 12: 463-518, 1996.
47. Chrzanowska-Wodnicka, M. and Burridge, K. Rho-stimulated contractility drives the formation of stress fibers and focal adhesions. J Cell Biol, 133: 1403-1415, 1996.
48. Kimura, K., Ito, M., Amano, M., Chihara, K., Fukata, Y., Nakafuku, M., Yamamori, B., Feng, J., Nakano, T., Okawa, K., Iwamatsu, A., and Kaibuchi, K. Regulation of myosin phosphatase by Rho and Rho-associated kinase (Rho-kinase). Science, 273: 245-248, 1996.
49. Kawano, Y., Fukata, Y., Oshiro, N., Amano, M., Nakamura, T., Ito, M., Matsumura, F., Inagaki, M., and Kaibuchi, K. Phosphorylation of myosin-binding subunit (MBS) of myosin phosphatase by Rho-kinase in vivo. J Cell Biol, 147: 1023-1038, 1999.
50. Kureishi, Y., Kobayashi, S., Amano, M., Kimura, K., Kanaide, H., Nakano, T., Kaibuchi, K., and Ito, M. Rho-associated kinase directly induces smooth muscle contraction through myosin light chain phosphorylation. J Biol Chem, 272: 12257-12260, 1997.
51. Amano, M., Chihara, K., Kimura, K., Fukata, Y., Nakamura, N., Matsuura, Y., and Kaibuchi, K. Formation of actin stress fibers and focal adhesions enhanced by Rho-kinase. Science, 275: 1308-1311, 1997.
52. Uehata, M., Ishizaki, T., Satoh, H., Ono, T., Kawahara, T., Morishita, T., Tamakawa, H., Yamagami, K., Inui, J., Maekawa, M., and Narumiya, S. Calcium sensitization of

smooth muscle mediated by a Rho-associated protein kinase in hypertension. Nature, 389: 990-994, 1997.
53. Riveline, D., Zamir, E., Balaban, N.Q., Schwarz, U.S., Ishizaki, T., Narumiya, S., Kam, Z., Geiger, B., and Bershadsky, A.D. Focal contacts as mechanosensors: externally applied local mechanical force induces growth of focal contacts by an mDia1-dependent and ROCK-independent mechanism. J Cell Biol, 153: 1175-1186, 2001.
54. Evers, E.E., Zondag, G.C., Malliri, A., Price, L.S., ten Klooster, J.P., van der Kammen, R.A., and Collard, J.G. Rho family proteins in cell adhesion and cell migration. Eur J Cancer, 36: 1269-1274, 2000.
55. Worthylake, R.A., Lemoine, S., Watson, J.M., and Burridge, K. RhoA is required for monocyte tail retraction during transendothelial migration. J Cell Biol, 154: 147-160, 2001.
56. Strauli, P. and Weiss, L. Cell locomation and tumor penetration. Report on a workshop of the EORTC cell surface project group. Eur J Cancer, 13: 1-12, 1977.
57. Strauli, P. and Haemmerli, G. The role of cancer cell motility in invasion. Cancer Metastasis Rev, 3: 127-141, 1984.
58. Trinkaus, J. Cells into Organs. Englewood Cliffs, NJ: Prentice Hall, Inc., 1984.
59. Wood, S. Pathogenesis of metastasis formation obsrved in vivo in the rabit ear chamber. Archives of Pathology, 66: 550, 1958.
60. Farina, K.L., Wyckoff, J.B., Rivera, J., Lee, H., Segall, J.E., Condeelis, J.S., and Jones, J.G. Cell motility of tumor cells visualized in living intact primary tumors using green fluorescent protein. Cancer Res, 58: 2528-2532, 1998.
61. Condeelis, J.S., Wyckoff, J., and Segall, J.E. Imaging of cancer invasion and metastasis using green fluorescent protein. Eur J Cancer, 36: 1671-1680, 2000.
62. Lackie, J.M. Cell movement and cell behaviour. London: Allen & Unwin, 1986.
63. Friedl, P. and Wolf, K. Tumour-cell invasion and migration: diversity and escape mechanisms. Nat Rev Cancer, 3: 362-374, 2003.
64. Verschueren, H., De Baetselier, P., and Bereiter-Hahn, J. Dynamic morphology of metastatic mouse T-lymphoma cells invading through monolayers of 10T1/2 cells. Cell Motil Cytoskeleton, 20: 203-214, 1991.
65. Kolega, J. The movement of cell clusters in vitro: morphology and directionality. J Cell Sci, 49: 15-32, 1981.
66. Friedl, P., Noble, P.B., Walton, P.A., Laird, D.W., Chauvin, P.J., Tabah, R.J., Black, M., and Zanker, K.S. Migration of coordinated cell clusters in mesenchymal and epithelial cancer explants in vitro. Cancer Res, 55: 4557-4560, 1995.
67. Knox, J.D., Cress, A.E., Clark, V., Manriquez, L., Affinito, K.S., Dalkin, B.L., and Nagle, R.B. Differential expression of extracellular matrix molecules and the alpha 6-integrins in the normal and neoplastic prostate. Am J Pathol, 145: 167-174, 1994.
68. Vandekerckhove, J., Leavitt, J., Kakunaga, T., and Weber, K. Coexpression of a mutant beta-actin and the two normal beta- and gamma-cytoplasmic actins in a stably transformed human cell line. Cell, 22: 893-899, 1980.
69. Sadano, H., Taniguchi, S., Kakunaga, T., and Baba, T. cDNA cloning and sequence of a new type of actin in mouse B16 melanoma. J Biol Chem, 263: 15868-15871, 1988.
70. Kaneda, A., Kaminishi, M., Sugimura, T., and Ushijima, T. Decreased expression of the seven ARP2/3 complex genes in human gastric cancers. Cancer Lett, 212: 203-210, 2004.
71. Otsubo, T., Iwaya, K., Mukai, Y., Mizokami, Y., Serizawa, H., Matsuoka, T., and Mukai, K. Involvement of Arp2/3 complex in the process of colorectal carcinogenesis. Mod Pathol, 17: 461-467, 2004.

72. Sossey-Alaoui, K., Ranalli, T.A., Li, X., Bakin, A.V., and Cowell, J.K. WAVE3 promotes cell motility and invasion through the regulation of MMP-1, MMP-3, and MMP-9 expression. Exp Cell Res, 308: 135-145, 2005.
73. Kurisu, S., Suetsugu, S., Yamazaki, D., Yamaguchi, H., and Takenawa, T. Rac-WAVE2 signaling is involved in the invasive and metastatic phenotypes of murine melanoma cells. Oncogene, 24: 1309-1319, 2005.
74. Lorenz, M., Yamaguchi, H., Wang, Y., Singer, R.H., and Condeelis, J. Imaging sites of N-wasp activity in lamellipodia and invadopodia of carcinoma cells. Curr Biol, 14: 697-703, 2004.
75. Yamaguchi, H., Lorenz, M., Kempiak, S., Sarmiento, C., Coniglio, S., Symons, M., Segall, J., Eddy, R., Miki, H., Takenawa, T., and Condeelis, J. Molecular mechanisms of invadopodium formation: the role of the N-WASP-Arp2/3 complex pathway and cofilin. J Cell Biol, 168: 441-452, 2005.
76. Yamaguchi, H., Miki, H., and Takenawa, T. Neural Wiskott-Aldrich syndrome protein is involved in hepatocyte growth factor-induced migration, invasion, and tubulogenesis of epithelial cells. Cancer Res, 62: 2503-2509, 2002.
77. Asch, H.L., Head, K., Dong, Y., Natoli, F., Winston, J.S., Connolly, J.L., and Asch, B.B. Widespread loss of gelsolin in breast cancers of humans, mice, and rats. Cancer Res, 56: 4841-4845, 1996.
78. Asch, H.L., Winston, J.S., Edge, S.B., Stomper, P.C., and Asch, B.B. Down-regulation of gelsolin expression in human breast ductal carcinoma in situ with and without invasion. Breast Cancer Res Treat, 55: 179-188, 1999.
79. Fujita, H., Okada, F., Hamada, J., Hosokawa, M., Moriuchi, T., Koya, R.C., and Kuzumaki, N. Gelsolin functions as a metastasis suppressor in B16-BL6 mouse melanoma cells and requirement of the carboxyl-terminus for its effect. Int J Cancer, 93: 773-780, 2001.
80. Lee, H.K., Driscoll, D., Asch, H., Asch, B., and Zhang, P.J. Downregulated gelsolin expression in hyperplastic and neoplastic lesions of the prostate. Prostate, 40: 14-19, 1999.
81. Tanaka, M., Sazawa, A., Shinohara, N., Kobayashi, Y., Fujioka, Y., Koyanagi, T., and Kuzumaki, N. Gelsolin gene therapy by retrovirus producer cells for human bladder cancer in nude mice. Cancer Gene Ther, 6: 482-487, 1999.
82. Thor, A.D., Edgerton, S.M., Liu, S., Moore, D.H., 2nd, and Kwiatkowski, D.J. Gelsolin as a negative prognostic factor and effector of motility in erbB-2-positive epidermal growth factor receptor-positive breast cancers. Clin Cancer Res, 7: 2415-2424, 2001.
83. De Corte, V., Bruyneel, E., Boucherie, C., Mareel, M., Vandekerckhove, J., and Gettemans, J. Gelsolin-induced epithelial cell invasion is dependent on Ras-Rac signaling. Embo J, 21: 6781-6790, 2002.
84. Zebda, N., Bernard, O., Bailly, M., Welti, S., Lawrence, D.S., and Condeelis, J.S. Phosphorylation of ADF/cofilin abolishes EGF-induced actin nucleation at the leading edge and subsequent lamellipod extension. J Cell Biol, 151: 1119-1128, 2000.
85. Yap, C.T., Simpson, T.I., Pratt, T., Price, D.J., and Maciver, S.K. The motility of glioblastoma tumour cells is modulated by intracellular cofilin expression in a concentration-dependent manner. Cell Motil Cytoskeleton, 60: 153-165, 2005.
86. Martoglio, A.M., Tom, B.D., Starkey, M., Corps, A.N., Charnock-Jones, D.S., and Smith, S.K. Changes in tumorigenesis- and angiogenesis-related gene transcript abundance profiles in ovarian cancer detected by tailored high density cDNA arrays. Mol Med, 6: 750-765, 2000.

87. Lee, S. and Helfman, D.M. Cytoplasmic p21Cip1 is involved in Ras-induced inhibition of the ROCK/LIMK/cofilin pathway. J Biol Chem, 279: 1885-1891, 2004.
88. Patel, AM., Incognito, L. S., Schechter, G. L., Wasilenko, W. J., and Somers, K. D. Amplification and expression of EMS-1 (cortactin) in head and neck squamous cell carcinoma cell lines. Oncogene, 12: 31-35, 1996.
89. Campbell, D. H., deFazio, A., Sutherland, R. L., and Daly, R. J. Expression and tyrosine phosphorylation of EMS1 in human breast cancer cell lines. Int J Cancer, 68: 485-492, 1996.
90. Chuma, M., Sakamoto, M., Yasuda, J., Fujii, G., Nakanishi, K., Tsuchiya, A., Ohta, T., Asaka, M., and Hirohashi, S. Overexpression of cortactin is involved in motility and metastasis of hepatocellular carcinoma. J Hepatol, 41: 629-636, 2004.
91. Bowden, E. T., Barth, M., Thomas, D., Glazer, R. I., and Mueller, S. C. An invasion-related complex of cortactin, paxillin and PKCmu associates with invadopodia at sites of extracellular matrix degradation. Oncogene, 18: 4440-4449, 1999.
92. Head, J. A., Jiang, D., Li, M., Zorn, L. J., Schaefer, E. M., Parsons, J. T., and Weed, S. A. Cortactin tyrosine phosphorylation requires Rac1 activity and association with the cortical actin cytoskeleton. Mol Biol Cell, 14: 3216-3229, 2003.
93. Timpson, P., Lynch, D. K., Schramek, D., Walker, F., and Daly, R. J. Cortactin overexpression inhibits ligand-induced down-regulation of the epidermal growth factor receptor. Cancer Res, 65: 3273-3280, 2005.
94. Lee, Y.G., Macoska, J.A., Korenchuk, S., and Pienta, K.J. MIM, a potential metastasis suppressor gene in bladder cancer. Neoplasia, 4: 291-294, 2002.
95. Lin, J., Liu, J., Wang, Y., Zhu, J., Zhou, K., Smith, N., and Zhan, X. Differential regulation of cortactin and N-WASP-mediated actin polymerization by missing in metastasis (MIM) protein. Oncogene, 24: 2059-2066, 2005.
96. Woodings, J.A., Sharp, S.J., and Machesky, L.M. MIM-B, a putative metastasis suppressor protein, binds to actin and to protein tyrosine phosphatase delta. Biochem J, 371: 463-471, 2003.
97. Mattila, P.K., Salminen, M., Yamashiro, T., and Lappalainen, P. Mouse MIM, a tissue-specific regulator of cytoskeletal dynamics, interacts with ATP-actin monomers through its C-terminal WH2 domain. J Biol Chem, 278: 8452-8459, 2003.
98. Sahai, E. and Marshall, C.J. RHO-GTPases and cancer. Nat Rev Cancer, 2: 133-142, 2002.
99. Ridley, A.J. Rho proteins and cancer. Breast Cancer Res Treat, 84: 13-19, 2004.
100. Wu, M., Wu, Z.F., Kumar-Sinha, C., Chinnaiyan, A., and Merajver, S.D. RhoC induces differential expression of genes involved in invasion and metastasis in MCF10A breast cells. Breast Cancer Res Treat, 84: 3-12, 2004.
101. van Golen, K.L., Wu, Z.F., Qiao, X.T., Bao, L.W., and Merajver, S.D. RhoC GTPase, a novel transforming oncogene for human mammary epithelial cells that partially recapitulates the inflammatory breast cancer phenotype. Cancer Res, 60: 5832-5838, 2000.
102. Clark, E.A., Golub, T.R., Lander, E.S., and Hynes, R.O. Genomic analysis of metastasis reveals an essential role for RhoC. Nature, 406: 532-535, 2000.
103. Kleer, C.G., Zhang, Y., Pan, Q., Gallagher, G., Wu, M., Wu, Z.F., and Merajver, S.D. WISP3 and RhoC guanosine triphosphatase cooperate in the development of inflammatory breast cancer. Breast Cancer Res, 6: R110-115, 2004.
104. Hakem, A., Sanchez-Sweatman, O., You-Ten, A., Duncan, G., Wakeham, A., Khokha, R., and Mak, T.W. RhoC is dispensable for embryogenesis and tumor initiation but essential for metastasis. Genes Dev, 19: 1974-1979, 2005.

105. Simpson, K.J., Dugan, A.S., and Mercurio, A.M. Functional analysis of the contribution of RhoA and RhoC GTPases to invasive breast carcinoma. Cancer Res, 64: 8694-8701, 2004.
106. van Golen, K.L., Bao, L., DiVito, M.M., Wu, Z., Prendergast, G.C., and Merajver, S.D. Reversion of RhoC GTPase-induced inflammatory breast cancer phenotype by treatment with a farnesyl transferase inhibitor. Mol Cancer Ther, 1: 575-583, 2002.
107. Adini, I., Rabinovitz, I., Sun, J.F., Prendergast, G.C., and Benjamin, L.E. RhoB controls Akt trafficking and stage-specific survival of endothelial cells during vascular development. Genes Dev, 17: 2721-2732, 2003.
108. Somlyo, A.V., Bradshaw, D., Ramos, S., Murphy, C., Myers, C.E., and Somlyo, A.P. Rho-kinase inhibitor retards migration and in vivo dissemination of human prostate cancer cells. Biochem Biophys Res Commun, 269: 652-659, 2000.
109. Jo, M., Thomas, K.S., Somlyo, A.V., Somlyo, A.P., and Gonias, S.L. Cooperativity between the Ras-ERK and Rho-Rho kinase pathways in urokinase-type plasminogen activator-stimulated cell migration. J Biol Chem, 277: 12479-12485, 2002.
110. Engers, R., Zwaka, T.P., Gohr, L., Weber, A., Gerharz, C.D., and Gabbert, H.E. Tiam1 mutations in human renal-cell carcinomas. Int J Cancer, 88: 369-376, 2000.
111. Engers, R., Springer, E., Michiels, F., Collard, J.G., and Gabbert, H.E. Rac affects invasion of human renal cell carcinomas by up-regulating tissue inhibitor of metalloproteinases (TIMP)-1 and TIMP-2 expression. J Biol Chem, 276: 41889-41897, 2001.
112. Peck, J., Douglas, G.t., Wu, C.H., and Burbelo, P.D. Human RhoGAP domain-containing proteins: structure, function and evolutionary relationships. FEBS Lett, 528: 27-34, 2002.
113. Wolf, R.M., Draghi, N., Liang, X., Dai, C., Uhrbom, L., Eklof, C., Westermark, B., Holland, E.C., and Resh, M.D. p190RhoGAP can act to inhibit PDGF-induced gliomas in mice: a putative tumor suppressor encoded on human chromosome 19q13.3. Genes Dev, 17: 476-487, 2003.
114. Wymann, M.P. and Marone, R. Phosphoinositide 3-kinase in disease: timing, location, and scaffolding. Curr Opin Cell Biol, 17: 141-149, 2005.
115. Zhou, H. and Kramer, R.H. Integrin engagement differentially modulates epithelial cell motility by RhoA/ROCK and PAK1. J Biol Chem, 280: 10624-10635, 2005.
116. Paszek, M.J., Zahir, N., Johnson, K.R., Lakins, J.N., Rozenberg, G.I., Gefen, A., Reinhart-King, C.A., Margulies, S.S., Dembo, M., Boettiger, D., Hammer, D.A., and Weaver, V.M. Tensional homeostasis and the malignant phenotype. Cancer Cell, 8: 241-254, 2005.
117. Rabinovitz, I., Gipson, I.K., and Mercurio, A.M. Traction forces mediated by alpha6beta4 integrin: implications for basement membrane organization and tumor invasion. Molecular Biology of the Cell, 12: 4030-4043, 2001.
118. Mercurio, A.M. and Rabinovitz, I. Towards a mechanistic understanding of tumor invasion--lessons from the alpha6beta 4 integrin. [Review] [103 refs]. Seminars in Cancer Biology, 11: 129-141, 2001.
119. Danen, E.H., van Rheenen, J., Franken, W., Huveneers, S., Sonneveld, P., Jalink, K., and Sonnenberg, A. Integrins control motile strategy through a Rho-cofilin pathway. J Cell Biol, 169: 515-526, 2005.
120. Chan, A.Y., Coniglio, S.J., Chuang, Y.Y., Michaelson, D., Knaus, U.G., Philips, M.R., and Symons, M. Roles of the Rac1 and Rac3 GTPases in human tumor cell invasion. Oncogene, 2005.

121. O'Connor, K.L. and Mercurio, A.M. Protein kinase A regulates Rac and is required for the growth factor-stimulated migration of carcinoma cells. Journal of Biological Chemistry, 276: 47895-47900, 2001.
122. O'Connor, K.L., Nguyen, B.K., and Mercurio, A.M. RhoA function in lamellae formation and migration is regulated by the alpha6beta4 integrin and cAMP metabolism. Journal of Cell Biology, 148: 253-258, 2000.
123. Wei, Q. and Adelstein, R.S. Pitx2a expression alters actin-myosin cytoskeleton and migration of HeLa cells through Rho GTPase signaling. Mol Biol Cell, 13: 683-697, 2002.
124. Wilkinson, S., Paterson, H.F., and Marshall, C.J. Cdc42-MRCK and Rho-ROCK signalling cooperate in myosin phosphorylation and cell invasion. Nat Cell Biol, 7: 255-261, 2005.

Chapter 5

CHARACTERIZATION OF THE FERM DOMAIN PROTEIN EHM2 IN HUMAN CANCER CELLS

Sanjay Chauhan[1], Ryan Childers[1], Jennifer Himes[1], Andrea Pierce[1], Sabrina Sykes[1], Kelvin W. Pond[3], Susan Kunz[1] and Roger L. Miesfeld[1,2]

[1]Departments of Biochemistry and Molecular Biophysics, [2]Molecular and Cellular Biology and the [3]Arizona Cancer Center, University of Arizona, Tucson, AZ, USA

Abstract: The FERM domain protein EHM2 (EPB41L4B) was first isolated and characterized based on its elevated expression in highly metastatic mouse melanoma cells. We recently found that human EHM2 is androgen-regulated in a cancer cell line model of steroid-induced cytoskeletal reorganization, and expression profiling analyses by others have shown that it is a primary steroid-regulated gene in rat liver and human lung cells. Bioinformatic analysis of human EHM2 revealed that it is a member of a unique subfamily of FERM domain proteins that includes the *Drosophila* YURT gene. Analysis of YURT protein functions in *Drosophila* have shown that it is required for dorsal closure during embryogenesis and is involved in mediating epithelial cell migration. We have used immunostaining to analyze steroid-induced and ectopic expression of EHM2 in the human fibrosarcoma cell line HT-1080 and found that it is localized to the cell membrane and associated with cytoskeletal reorganization. We have also found that EHM2 is highly expressed in the metastatic prostate cancer cell lines LNCaP, DU-145 and PC-3 cells, and moreover, that EHM2 transcripts are present at significantly higher levels in human prostate tumors than in non-malignant prostate cells. Based on these data, we propose that elevated expression of EHM2 may enhance the metastatic properties of advanced prostate cancers.

Key words: EPB41L4B; cell migration; dihydrotestosterone; prostate cancer; LNCaP

A.E. Cress and R.B. Nagle (eds.), Cell Adhesion and Cytoskeletal Molecules in Metastasis, 91–102.

1. EHM2 IS A MEMBER OF THE FERM DOMAIN FAMILY OF CYTOSKELETAL PROTEINS

Cancer biologists have long studied cytoskeletal reorganization and cell attachment to extracellular matrices to determine the mechanisms that control metastatic potential (1, 2). Proteins involved in coordinating events at the plasma membrane through protein interaction domains or modules have been identified using molecular genetic and biochemical approaches. One such family of proteins are those containing a FERM (Four.1 protein, Ezrin, Radixin, Moesin) domain which functions as a protein docking surface with the cytosolic tail of transmembrane proteins such as CD44 (3). The molecular structures of several FERM domain proteins have been solved (4-6) and these data reveal that FERM domains consist of a three lobes (F1, F2, F3) which together form a protein binding surface. The F1 and F2 domains are the most highly conserved amongst all FERM domain proteins, and the F3 domain has been shown to encode binding sites that contribute to target protein specificity (6).

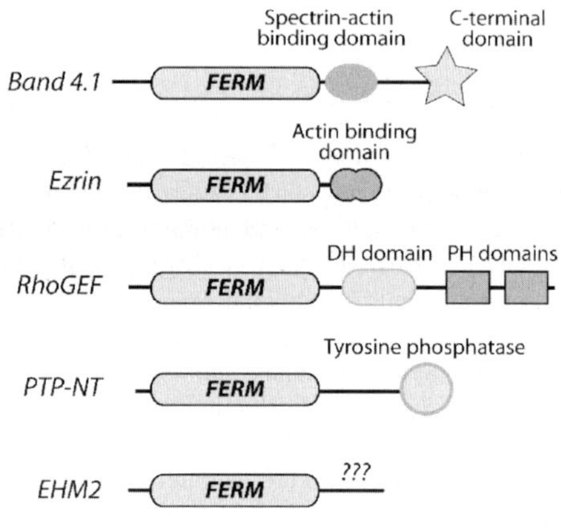

Figure 1. Functional organization of representative FERM domain proteins. The FERM domain is a conserved ~300 amino acid sequence found in numerous proteins associated with the cytoskeleton. The Band 4.1 and ezrin proteins are the best characterized and function as "tethers" that link the cytoskeleton to the cytoplasmic domain of membrane proteins. The Rho-GEF (guanine nucleotide exchange factor) and PTP-NT (protein tyrosine phosphatase) FERM domain proteins are thought to function as targeted signaling proteins that associate with the plasma membrane. Bioinformatic analysis of the EHM2 coding sequence does not reveal any protein motifs outside of the FERM domain.

The FERM domain contains ~300 amino acids (7), and is represented by a large family of highly conserved proteins belonging to 11 distinct subfamilies based on bioinformatic analysis (8). As shown in Figure 1, most FERM domain proteins contain an N-terminal FERM domain that is linked to one or more C-terminal components encoding an actin binding domain, a protein tyrosine phosphatase, or even a Rho guanine nucleotide exchange factor (GEF) function (3, 9). One of the best characterized FERM domain proteins is ezrin which has recently been shown to be over-expressed in advanced stage human rhabdomyosarcomas and required for Rho-mediated signaling in a metastatic rhabdomyosarcoma cell model (10). Ezrin is also expressed and androgen-regulated in prostate cells (11), although it is not known if ezrin contributes to metastasis in prostate cancer.

We are interested in steroid-regulation of cancer cell phenotypes and recently developed a model to investigate androgen control of cytoskeletal organization using the human fibrosarcoma cell line HT-1080 (8, 12). We discovered that reconstitution of androgen receptor (AR) expression in a subclone of HT-1080 cells called HT-AR1, uniquely induces growth arrest, cytoskeletal reorganization, and neuroendocrine-like cell differentiation. Expression profiling analyses revealed that androgen treatment of HT-AR1 cells with dihydrotestosterone (DHT) leads to coordinate expression of numerous genes associated with cytoskeletal reorganization, including EHM2 (13), RhoB (14), PTGF-β (15), caveolin-2 (16), Egr-1 (17), and myosin 1B (18). While it is possible that each of these genes contributes to the observed androgen response, we were particularly interested in EHM2 because the mouse ortholog had previously been reported by Shimizu et al. (19) to be associated with cell metastasis. In addition, EHM2 has recently been shown to be a primary glucocorticoid-regulated gene in a human lung cancer cell line (20) and rat liver cells (21), suggesting that androgen regulation in HT-AR1 cells is a direct effect of AR.

Unlike most FERM domain proteins that contain a second functional domain in the C-terminal region, EHM2 lacks such signature sequences based on extensive bioinformatic analysis (Figure 1). This suggests that EHM2 either encodes a novel activity, or perhaps, functions as a dominant negative modulator of other FERM domain proteins. Since FERM domain proteins have been implicated in cytoskeletal organization and cell motility (3, 7, 13), we characterized the expression of the human EHM2 gene in the HT-AR1 cell model (8). We found that DHT treatment results in rapid induction of a 3.8 kb transcript that encodes a protein of 504 amino acids, and moreover, that this same transcript is present in human testes, prostate and breast tissue. The *Drosophila* ortholog of EHM2 called YURT, has also been characterized (13) and shown to be localized to the apical and lateral domains of the plasma membrane and involved in epithelial cell migration. Genetic analysis demonstrated that YURT is required for dorsal closure during embryogenesis and that loss-of-function mutations are embryonic lethal. Consistent with these findings, the murine EHM2 gene is expressed during days 7-17 of embryogenesis at a time when tissue development is critical (19).

2. DIHYDROTESTOSTERONE TREATMENT OF HT-AR1 CELLS STIMULATES CELL MIGRATION

Our finding that DHT treatment of HT-AR1 cells induces growth arrest and neuroendocrine-like cell differentiation, suggests that HT-1080 cells may have been derived from a stem cell cancer (8). To better characterize this steroidal response at the cellular level, we used time lapse videomicroscopy to record cell movement over a five hour period in the presence and absence of DHT. Surprisingly, these analyses revealed that DHT treatment induced rapid changes in cell morphology and migration (12). We have now used this time lapse videomicroscopy data to quantitatively determine the movement of individual cells under the two different culture conditions. As shown in Figure 2, DHT treatment induced a significant increase in cell migration, suggesting that androgen-regulated gene expression results in altered cell migratory properties in this cancer cell model.

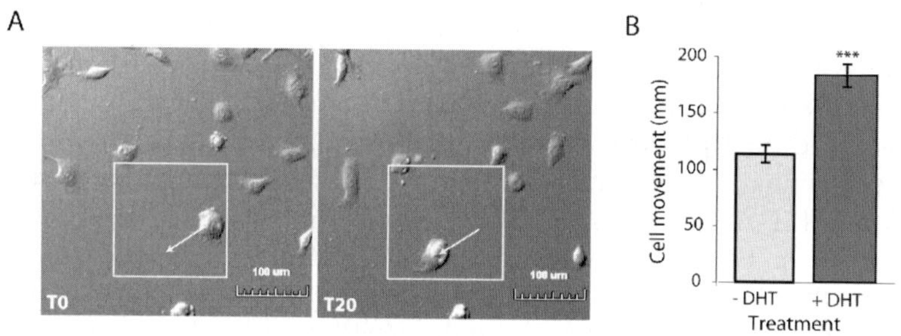

Figure 2. Dihydrotestosterone treatment of HT-AR1 cells induces cell migration. Time lapse videomicroscopy was used to measure cell migration in HT-AR1 cell cultures treated with steroid for five hours (10 nM DHT). A) Representative pictures taken 20 minutes apart showing the migration of a single cell as highlighted by the arrow. Images were captured using a grayscale CCD camera mounted on an inverted Olympus IMT2 microscope equipped with a BiopTechs Delta T live cell system (Bioptechs, Inc. Butler, PA.). B) Quantitation of cell migration in HT-AR1 cell cultures as a function of DHT treatment. Cell migration was measured using SimplePCI 4.0 software (Compix Imaging Inc, Cranberry Township, PA.) to track the movement of twenty cells over a five hour period and the mean and standard deviation of cell movement (in mm) is shown. Statistical analysis revealed that DHT treatment caused a significant increase in HT-AR1 cell migration over this time period as shown by the asterisks ($p<0.0001$).

3. EXPRESSION OF EHM2 PROTEIN IS ASSOCIATED WITH CYTOSKELETAL REORGANIZATION

We characterized EHM2 protein expression in HT-AR1 cells using polyclonal antibodies directed against the unique C-terminal region. For these experiments, a polypeptide of 150 amino acids corresponding to the unique portion of the F3 subdomain and 100 amino acids beyond the FERM domain, was produced in bacteria and used as an antigen to generate rabbit polyclonal antibodies. As shown in Figure 3, EHM2 immunostaining of HT-AR1 cells cultured on fibronectin-coated coverslips in the presence or absence of DHT showed a dramatic increase in EHM2 protein expression that was associated with the cell membrane. The punctate pattern of EHM2 staining was most pronounced in cells that had undergone cytoskeletal reorganization and was consistent with localization of this FERM domain protein to the cell membrane. We also observed an increase in nuclear staining in DHT-treated cells, although the basis for this is unknown and could reflect cross-reactivity of the antibody.

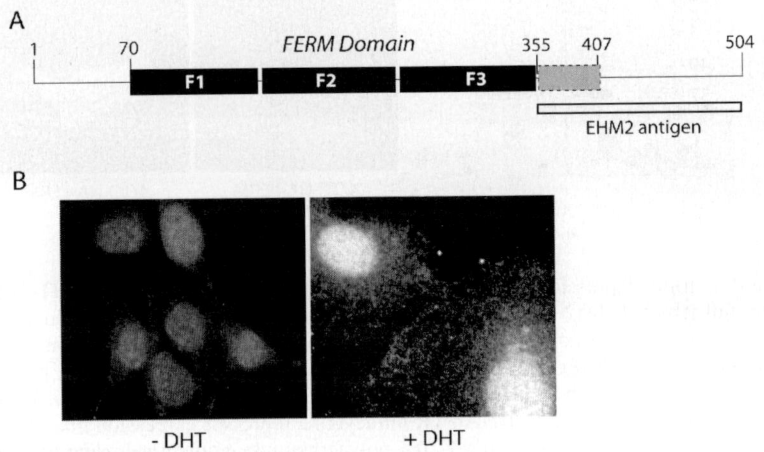

Figure 3. Androgen-induction of EHM2 protein expression in HT-AR1 cells. A) A rabbit polyclonal antibody was generated using a 150 amino acid polypeptide derived from the C-terminal region of human EHM2 which includes ~50 amino acids of the extended F3 domain. B) Immunostaining of HT-AR1 cells cultured on fibronectin-coated coverslips for three days in the presence or absence of 10 nM DHT. Representative fluorescent images are shown. Note that the punctate staining pattern of EHM2 was associated primarily with cells that had undergone cytoskeletal reorganization.

In order to investigate the structure and function of EHM2 independent of androgen signaling, we cloned the full-length EHM2 coding sequence into the tetracycline-regulated expression vector pcDNA4/TO (p4/TO) and attached the FLAG epitope sequence to the N-terminus. Transient transfection of HT-AR1 cells with either the p4/TO vector alone, the recombinant p4/TO -FLAG-EHM2 expression vector, or the p4/TO-FLAG-EHM2 expression vector in the presence of the pcDNA6/TR tetracycline

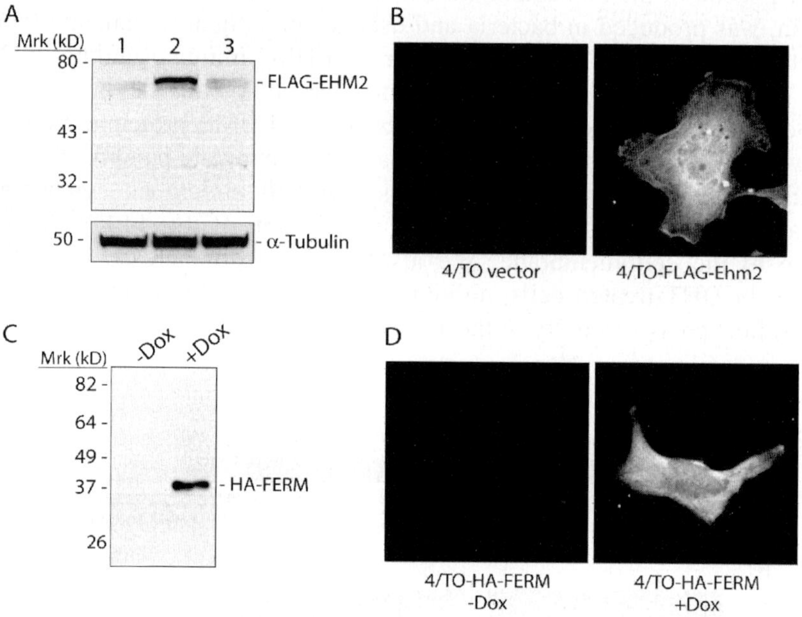

Figure 4. Ectopic expression of epitope-tagged EHM2 protein in transfected HT-1080 cells. A) The full-length EHM2 coding sequence containing a FLAG epitope sequence at the N-terminus was cloned into the pcDNA4/TO tetracycline-regulated expression vector and transfected into HT-1080 cells. Protein extracts from cells transfected with the pcDNA4/TO vector alone (lane 1), the pcDNA4/TO-EHM2 plasmid (lane 2), or co-transfected with pcDNA4/TO-EHM2 and the pcDNA6/TR tetracycline repressor expression plasmid (lane 3), were analyzed by Western blots on a 4-20% polyacrylamide gradient gel using an anti-FLAG antibody. The location of the ~58 kD molecular weight FLAG-EHM2 protein is shown. B) Transfection of HT-1080 cells with the p4/TO vector alone or the p4/TO-EHM2 plasmid and analyzed by immunostaining using anti-FLAG antibodies. C) Western blot of protein extracts made from HT-TR71 cells (HT-1080 cells stably expressing the tetracycline repressor protein) grown in the presence or absence of doxycycline (Dox) following transfection with a p4/TO expression plasmid containing the 350 amino acid FERM domain of EHM2 (p4/TO-HA-FERM) linked to the hemagglutinin (HA) epitope sequence at the N-terminus. The expected Dox-induced ~40 kD HA-FERM domain EHM2 protein is shown. D) Anti-HA immunostaining of HT-TR71 cells transfected with p4/TO-HA-FERM and cultured in the presence or absence Dox.

repressor plasmid, confirmed that the EHM2 coding sequence directed the expression of the full-length protein based on western blotting with anti-FLAG antibodies (Figure 4). Moreover, immunostaining of transiently transfected cells with anti-FLAG antibody showed that FLAG-EHM2 expression was associated with the cell membrane, similar to the pattern seen using EHM2 antibodies to analyze HT-AR1 cells treated with DHT.

We also constructed an EHM2 expression vector in p4/TO containing the extended 350 amino acid FERM domain, and in this case, linked two copies of the hemagglutinin epitope tag (HA) to the N-terminus. Transient transfection of HT-1080 cells that had been stably-transfected with the p6/TR tetracycline repressor plasmid (HT-TR71 cells), showed that doxycycline treatment induced the expression of the expected ~40 kDa HA-FERM protein. Immunostaining of transfected HT-TR71 cells cultured in the presence or absence of doxycycline for 48 hours demonstrated that this truncated EHM2 protein behaved similarly to the full-length protein. Studies are currently underway to isolate stable HT-TR71 transfectants that express either the full-length FLAG-EHM2 or HA-FERM proteins under doxycycline control in order to investigate the role of EHM2 in cytoskeletal reorganization and cell migration.

4. HUMAN PROSTATE CANCER CELL LINES CONTAIN HIGH LEVELS OF EHM2 TRANSCRIPTS

Since EHM2 is a steroid-regulated gene in several different cell types (8, 20, 21), and has been associated with metastasis in melanoma cells (19), we wondered if EHM2 might be expressed at elevated levels in prostate cancer cells. For these studies, we used quantitative real-time RT-PCR to analyze EHM2 transcript levels in the three metastatic human prostate cancer cell lines, LNCaP, DU-145 and PC-3, and compared this to EHM2 levels in a human eosinophilic leukemia cell line, EOL-1, and in HT-1080 cells. As shown in Figure 5, all three of the prostate cancer cell lines had higher levels of EHM2 transcripts than either HT-1080 or EOL-1 cells, with LNCaP cells having the highest amounts. Interestingly, both PC-3 and DU-145 cells do not express the androgen receptor, suggesting that EHM2 expression is androgen-independent in these cells. Since the cell lines were cultured in media containing 10% calf serum, rather than steroid-free media, it is possible that corticosteroids in the serum could be activating EHM2 expression through the glucocorticoid receptor (20, 21). It is also likely that in addition to androgens, other growth promoting signals activate EHM2 expression in prostate cancer cells.

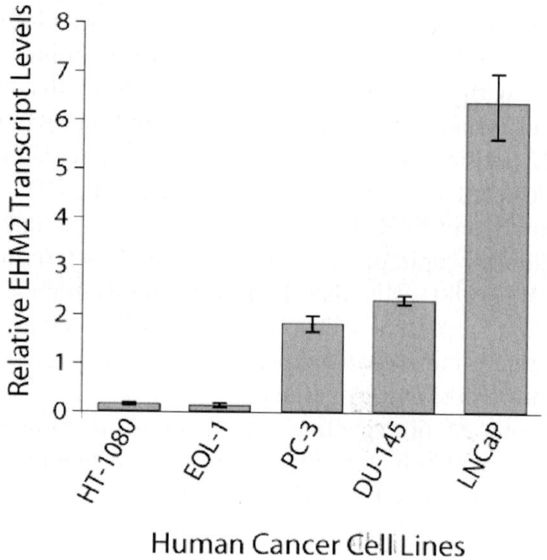

Figure 5. Quantitation of EHM2 transcript levels in prostate cancer cell lines. Real-time RT-PCR was performed on the ABI Prism 7000 sequence detection system (Applied Biosystems, Foster City, CA) using ABI primers for EHM2 (Hs00298360) and GAPDH (Hs99999905). Based on the results of triplicate experiments using total RNA isolated from each cell line, the PCR efficiency was calculated according to Ramakers et al. (27) and target gene ratios relative to GAPD gene expression were calculated using the method of Pfaffl et al. (28). The mean +/- standard error of the mean for each cell sample is shown.

5. DATABASE MINING REVEALS HIGH LEVELS OF EHM2 TRANSCRIPTS IN PROSTATE CANCER

To determine if EHM2 transcript levels differ between normal tissues and the corresponding cancer cell types, we took advantage of the Oncomine database analysis tool developed by Chinnaiyan and colleagues (22, 23). At the time of analysis, the Oncomine database (http://www.oncomine.org) contained 90 datasets from 6,372 microarrays which were queried for the expression of EHM2 (EPB41L4B) using the online analysis tool. Statistically significant differences (adjusted P-values <0.05) were found in four matched datasets from liver, pancreas, lung and prostate cells. We found that EHM2 transcript levels were significantly increased in prostate cancer samples compared to normal or non-malignant prostate samples, whereas, EHM2 transcript levels were higher in normal liver, pancreatic and lung tissue samples as compared to cancer tissue samples. Oncomine analysis of the expression profiling data from the three prostate studies used in this comparison are shown in Figure 6. Study 1 had an adjusted P-value of 4.1×10^{-5} based on comparing EHM2 transcript levels in 16 BPH and 6 normal prostate samples to that of 59 primary prostate cancer samples (24). Study 2 compared 15 normal prostate samples with 15 adjacent prostate cancer samples (25) and had an adjusted P-value of 0.04. Lastly, study 3 compared 9 BPH samples with 16 prostate cancer samples (26) and had an adjusted P-value of 0.003. Importantly, a similar query of EHM2 transcript levels in SAGE datasets from the Cancer Genome Anatomy Project (http://cgap.nci.nih.gov), confirmed that EHM2 is expressed at higher levels in prostate cancer cells as compared to normal prostate tissue (data not shown).

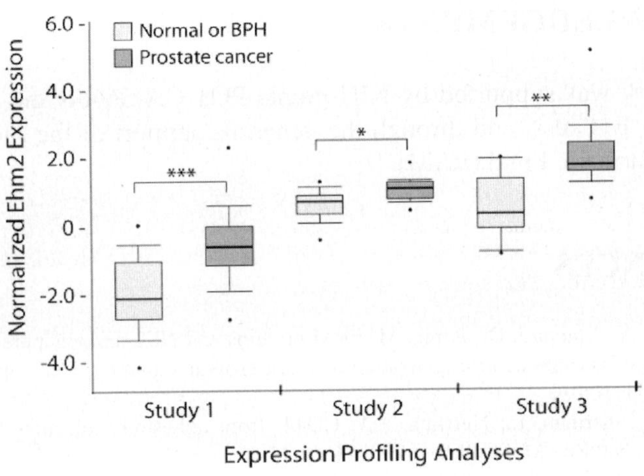

Figure 6. EHM2 transcript levels are elevated in human prostate cancer cells. Database mining was performed using the Oncomine database analysis tool (http://www.oncomine.org) developed by Chinnaiyan and colleagues (22, 23). The adjusted P-values for each dataset were 4.1×10^{-5} for study 1 (24), 0.04 for study 2 (25) and 0.003 for study 3 (26).

6. SUMMARY

Steroid-regulation of cytoskeletal organization and cell migration is most often associated with developmental processes occurring during embryogenesis. However, in cancer cell types that respond to steroid signaling such as breast and prostate cancer, hormonal signals may also play a role in cell metastasis. For example, steroid signaling in cancer stem cells could alter the expression of genes normally involved in cell migration during development and thereby enhance the metastatic potential of these cells. The finding that FERM domain proteins such as ezrin (10) and EHM2 (19) are over-expressed in metastatic cancers, and that both of these proteins are androgen-regulated (8, 11), suggest that they could contribute to prostate cancer progression by altering cytoskeletal structures in response to steroids. Clearly, future studies are warranted to better understand the role of FERM domain proteins such as ezrin and EHM2 in cancer cell metastasis.

ACKNOWLEDGEMENTS

This work was supported by NIH grants PO1 CA 56666 and CA 75152 to Dr. Anne E. Cress, and through the generous support of the Jack Findlay Doyle II Charitable Fund (RLM).

REFERENCES

1. Gautreau, A., Louvard, D., Arpin, M. ERM proteins and NF2 tumor suppressor: the Yin and Yang of cortical actin organization and cell growth signaling. Curr Opin Cell Biol 2002, 14(1): 104-9.
2. Ponta, H., Sherman, L., Herrlich, P.A. CD44: from adhesion molecules to signalling regulators. Nat Rev Mol Cell Biol 2003, 4(1): 33-45.
3. Sun, C.X., Robb, V.A., Gutmann, D.H. Protein 4.1 tumor suppressors: getting a FERM grip on growth regulation. J Cell Sci 2002, 115(Pt 21): 3991-4000.
4. Hamada, K., Shimizu, T., Yonemura, S, Tsukita, S, Hakoshima, T. Structural basis of adhesion-molecule recognition by ERM proteins revealed by the crystal structure of the radixin-ICAM-2 complex. Embo J 2003, 22(3): 502-14.
5. Shimizu, T., Seto, A., Maita, N., Hamada, K., Tsukita, S., Hakoshima, T. Structural basis for neurofibromatosis type 2. Crystal structure of the merlin FERM domain. J Biol Chem 2002, 277(12): 10332-6.
6. Smith, W.J., Nassar, N., Bretscher, A., Cerione, R.A., Karplus, P.A. Structure of the Active N-terminal Domain of Ezrin. J Biol Chem 2003, 278(7): 4949-56.
7. Chishti, A.H., Kim, A.C., Marfatia, S.M., et al. The FERM domain: a unique module involved in the linkage of cytoplasmic proteins to the membrane. Trends Biochem Sci 1998, 23(8): 281-2.

8. Chauhan, S., Pandey, R., Way, J., et al. Androgen regulation of the human FERM domain encoding gene EHM2 in a cell model of steroid-induced differentiation. Biochem Biophys Res Commun 2003, 310: 421-32.
9. Kubo, T., Yamashita, T., Yamaguchi, A., Sumimoto, H., Hosokawa, K., Tohyama, M. A novel FERM domain including guanine nucleotide exchange factor is involved in Rac signaling and regulates neurite remodeling. J Neurosci 2002, 2(19): 8504-13.
10. Yu, Y., Khan, J., Khanna, C., Helman, L., Meltzer, P.S., Merlino, G. Expression profiling identifies the cytoskeletal organizer ezrin and the developmental homeoprotein Six-1 as key metastatic regulators. Nat Med 2004, 10(2): 175-81.
11. Pang, S.T., Dillner, K., Wu, X., Pousette, A., Norstedt, G., Flores-Morales, A. Gene expression profiling of androgen deficiency predicts a pathway of prostate apoptosis that involves genes related to oxidative stress. Endocrinology 2002, 143(12): 4897-906.
12. Chauhan, S., Kunz, S., Davis, K., et al. Androgen control of cell proliferation and cytoskeletal reorganization in human fibrosarcoma cells: role of RhoB signaling. J Biol Chem 2004, 279(2): 937-44.
13. Hoover, K.B., Bryant, P.J. Drosophila Yurt is a new protein-4.1-like protein required for epithelial morphogenesis. Dev Genes Evol 2002, 212(5): 230-8.
14. Liu, J.P., Jessell, T.M. A role for rhoB in the delamination of neural crest cells from the dorsal neural tube. Development 1998, 125(24): 5055-67.
15. Li, P.X., Wong, J., Ayed, A., et al. Placental transforming growth factor-beta is a downstream mediator of the growth arrest and apoptotic response of tumor cells to DNA damage and p53 overexpression. J Biol Chem 2000, 275(26): 20127-35.
16. Razani B., Wang, X.B., Engelman, J.A., et al. Caveolin-2-deficient mice show evidence of severe pulmonary dysfunction without disruption of caveolae. Mol Cell Biol 2002, 22(7): 2329-44.
17. Russell, D.L., Doyle, K.M., Gonzales-Robayna, I., Pipaon, C., Richards, J.S. Egr-1 induction in rat granulosa cells by follicle-stimulating hormone and luteinizing hormone: combinatorial regulation by transcription factors cyclic adenosine 3',5'-monophosphate regulatory element binding protein, serum response factor, sp1, and early growth response factor-1. Mol Endocrinol 2003, 17(4): 520-33.
18. Raposo, G., Cordonnier, M.N., Tenza, D., et al. Association of myosin I alpha with endosomes and lysosomes in mammalian cells. Mol Biol Cell 1999, 10(5): 1477-94.
19. Shimizu, K., Nagamachi, Y., Tani, M., et al. Molecular cloning of a novel NF2/ERM/4.1 superfamily gene, ehm2, that is expressed in high-metastatic K1735 murine melanoma cells. Genomics 2000, 65(2): 113-20.
20. Wang, J.C., Derynck, M.K., Nonaka, D.F., Khodabakhsh, D.B., Haqq, C., Yamamoto, K.R. Chromatin immunoprecipitation (ChIP) scanning identifies primary glucocorticoid receptor target genes. Proc Natl Acad Sci U S A 2004, 101(44): 15603-8.
21. Phuc, Le P., Friedman, J.R., Schug, J., et al. Glucocorticoid Receptor-Dependent Gene Regulatory Networks. PLoS Genet 2005, 1(2): e16.
22. Rhodes, D.R., Yu, J., Shanker, K., et al. Large-scale meta-analysis of cancer microarray data identifies common transcriptional profiles of neoplastic transformation and progression. Proc Natl Acad Sci U S A 2004, 101(25): 9309-14.
23. Rhodes, D.R., Yu, J., Shanker, K., et al. ONCOMINE: a cancer microarray database and integrated data-mining platform. Neoplasia 2004, 6(1): 1-6.
24. Dhanasekaran, S.M., Barrette, T.R., Ghosh, D., et al. Delineation of prognostic biomarkers in prostate cancer. Nature 2001, 412(6849): 822-6.
25. Luo, J.H., Yu, Y.P., Cieply, K., et al. Gene expression analysis of prostate cancers. Mol Carcinog 2002, 33(1): 25-35.

26. Luo, J., Duggan, D.J., Chen, Y., et al. Human prostate cancer and benign prostatic hyperplasia: molecular dissection by gene expression profiling. Cancer Res 2001, 61(12): 4683-8.
27. Ramakers, C., Ruijter, J.M., Deprez, R.H., Moorman, A.F. Assumption-free analysis of quantitative real-time polymerase chain reaction (PCR) data. Neurosci Lett 2003, 339(1): 62-6.
28. Pfaffl, M.W. A new mathematical model for relative quantification in real-time RT-PCR. Nucleic Acids Res 2001, 29(9): e45.

Chapter 6

CYTOKERATIN 6 EXPRESSION IN PROSTATE STEM CELLS

Monika Schmelz[1,2] and Anil Prasad [1,2]
[1]*Department of Pathology, Southern Arizona Veterans Affairs Health Care System, Tucson, AZ, USA,* [2]*Department of Pathology, Arizona Health Sciences Center, University of Arizona, Tucson, AZ, USA*

Abstract: The simplified epithelium of the human prostate gland is representative of a slowly growing but morphologically dynamic tissue. The normal prostate gland contains, in part, the persistent basal cell population and the putative stem cells. It has been postulated by others that the transformation of normal glandular structures into cancer glands and subsequent tumor progression may involve aberrant regulation of the stem cell population. In this chapter, the induction of cytokeratin 6 expression is postulated to participate in the transition of a stem cell from its specialized niche within the basal cell population into a differentiated state. The basic morphological features of the normal prostate gland are reviewed and the molecular features of the prostate stem cells are discussed. Data is presented to illustrate the defining features of a new epithelial phenotype in the prostate gland, containing both cytokeratin 6 expression and the capability to differentiate and reach from the basal cell layer to the luminal surface of the gland. These results underscore the plasticity of the epithelial cell layers and the potential for cytokeratin 6 to serve as an efficient marker for an important subset of the basal cell population. Further investigation will be required in animal models to determine the essential nature of the cytokeratin 6 expression for the normal development of the prostate gland.

Key words: epithelium; cytokeratin 6; prostate; gland; basal cells; luminal cells; development; human prostate glands; stem cells; zonula occludens

A.E. Cress and R.B. Nagle (eds.), Cell Adhesion and Cytoskeletal Molecules in Metastasis, 103–122.

1. PROSTATE CANCER: THE CLINICAL PROBLEM

Adenocarcinoma of the prostate is the most common form of cancer in men and the second leading cause of morbidity and cancer death (1). In 2003, about 220,900 new cases were diagnosed, of which approximately 29,000 may progress to lethality. Cancer of the prostate is typically a disease of older men (age > 50 years). The age adjusted incidence of prostate cancer in USA is 69/100,000. There are some remarkable and inexplicable national and racial differences in the incidence of this disease (2). Prostate cancer is not common among Asians. Age-adjusted incidence among Asians is 2-3/100,000 compared with a rate of 50-60 among US Caucasians. However, prostate cancer is more prevalent among the African-American population.

Prostate cancer is a disorder of cell differentiation and cell proliferation with unknown cause. One hypothesis (3) is based on histopathological observations of abnormal morphological prostatic growth in young adults including the asynchronous postpubertal and fetal development of the prostate (4). This hypothesis proposes that the origins of prostatic diseases, including carcinoma, are to be found in the *in utero* influences of the developing prostate (3). Three other theories have been proposed (5). The first theory is that the changes in the ratios of androgens and/or estrogens with age stimulate prostate cell growth. The second is that alterations in epithelial-mesenchymal interactions, through a stimulation of the embryonic inductive potential of the stroma, lead to an increase in proliferation. The third suggests that there is an expansion of an epithelial stem cell population.

Stem cells have not yet been definitively identified within the prostate, since there are currently no specific markers for prostate epithelial stem cells. The identification and characterization of stem cells in prostate tissue is widely considered as very important, because these cells may represent major targets of carcinogenesis. An understanding of prostatic epithelial biology including the location and characteristics of prostatic stem cells is also important, because the evolution of androgen-independent prostate carcinoma, a feature of tumor progression, may reflect a stem cell-like state of the tumor (6).

2. THE ADULT NORMAL PROSTATE GLAND: A SPECIAL GLANDULAR STRUCTURE

The normal and hyperplastic prostatic epithelium consists of two histologically defined cellular compartments, the basal layer and the secretory layer surrounded by a basal lamina. A third cell type, the neuroendocrine cells, is rare, and scattered throughout the basal and luminal compartments in the acini and ducts (7).

Basal cells are androgen independent and can be distinguished from luminal cells by their unique expression of cytokeratins 5/14/15/17 and CD 44 (8), and lack of expression of the prostate specific antigen (PSA). Another characteristic of the basal cell layer is the expression of Bcl-2, which usually blocks apoptosis in stem cells and other proliferating, self-renewal compartments (9). The basal cell layer represents the proliferative compartment and most probably houses the prostatic stem cell population. Recent data on the immunolocalization of nuclear androgen receptor in the human prostate have indicated that basal cells can be potentially and focally androgen receptive, most likely those which may give rise to secretory luminal cells (10). In contrast, the secretory luminal cells are androgen dependent and express predominantly cytokeratins 8 and 18 (11), PSA and prostatic acid phosphatase (PAP). The basal membrane surrounding the prostate gland is composed of collagen IV, collagen VII, entactin, variable amounts of fibronectin, vitronectin and tenascin and the laminin subchains $\alpha1$, $\alpha2$, $\beta1$, $\beta2$, $\gamma1$ as well as $\beta3\alpha3\gamma2$ subchains of laminin 5 (12) and Laminin 10 (13). The adhesion between epithelial cells and the basement membrane as well as cell-cell adhesion is considered to play an important role in directing epithelial cell polarity and differentiation into functional tissues (14).

In the normal prostatic gland, two major adhesion structures mediate the cell to extracellular matrix (ECM) adhesion: the hemidesmosomes and the focal contacts (12). Hemidesmosomes (HD's) are specialized morphological structures that mediate the adhesion of basal epithelial cells to the basal lamina in stratified and certain complex epithelia such as the prostate gland. HD's provide links between the cytokeratin intermediate filaments (IF's) and the extracellular matrix. HD's are composed of a number of distinct proteins including the $\alpha6\beta4$ integrins, HD1, BP180, BP230, IFAP300 and plectin. The non-covalently associated integrin heterodimer $\alpha6\beta4$ is a transmembrane protein, which is considered to be responsible for the integration of the cytoskeleton and the extracellular matrix at the hemidesmosomal structure (15). Focal contacts are dynamic, heterogeneous structures in which transmembrane adhesion receptors (integrins) provide a structural link between the actin cytoskeleton and the extracellular matrix components.

There is strong evidence that the stroma has influence on the differentiation of glandular structures in the prostate (16). However, the basic processes of the maintenance of tissue homeostasis, the balance between differentiation and growth, in the human prostate are still very poorly elucidated.

3. ALTERATION OF THE BASAL CELL COMPARTMENT IN EARLY CANCER PROGRESSION

PIN, referred to as high grade prostatic intraepithelial neoplasia, is considered as the precursor of prostatic adenocarcinoma. There is substantial evidence linking PIN and cancer (17-19). Firstly, the incidence and extent of PIN and cancer increase with patient age. Secondly, PIN and cancer are usually multiclonal and multifocal (17-21). Thirdly, the peripheral zone of the prostate, the area in which the majority of prostatic carcinomas occur (70%), is also the most common location for PIN (19, 22). The continuum which culminates in high grade PIN and early invasive cancer is characterized by progressive basal cell layer disruption, abnormalities in markers of secretory differentiation, and genetic instability (23-27).

Increasing grades of PIN are associated with progressive disruption of the basal cell layer. The amount of disruption increases with increasing grades of PIN, with loss of more than one-third of the basal cell layer in 52% of foci of high grade PIN (22). Early events in invasive carcinoma occur as glandular out-pouching from areas with basal cell disruption (19, 22).

In PIN lesions, neoplastic cells gradually replace the normal luminal secretory epithelium and a progressive alteration of the basal cell layer and basal membrane disruption occurs. In neoplastic glands the basal cells are altered and with them, essential hemidesmosomal structures that define the gland. Except for α6 and α3, integrins in general are downregulated and β4 integrin, laminin 5 and other hemidesmosomal adhesive molecules are not expressed in prostate cancer (28). Figures 1 and 2 show some of the molecular changes that occur during prostate cancer progression.

Recently, three different prostate tumor phenotypes were distinguished based on differential integrin expression, one possibly being indicative of a more invasive behavior (29). In addition, a new variant of adhesion complex, which contained CD 151, was described in prostate tumors (29). Hemidesmosome structures are important for the maintenance of normal glandular architecture and the loss of these structures may be significant for the loss of basal cell differentiation in tumor progression.

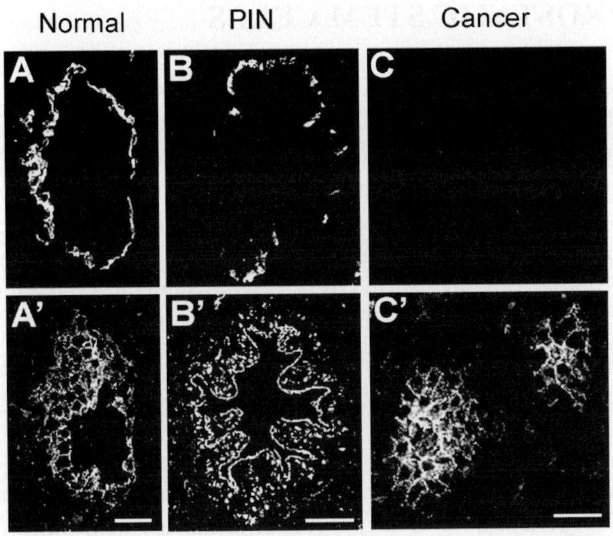

Figure 1. Immunofluorescence doublestaining of the prostatic basal cell marker cytokeratin 5 (A,B,C) with desmoplakin (A',C') and with the tight junctional protein ZO-1 (B') in a normal prostate gland (A,A'), in prostatic intraepithelial neoplasia (PIN; B,B') and in cancerous gland (C, C'). Note the partial lack of basal cells in the PIN lesions and the complete lack of basal cells within the carcinoma. Bars, 30 μm.

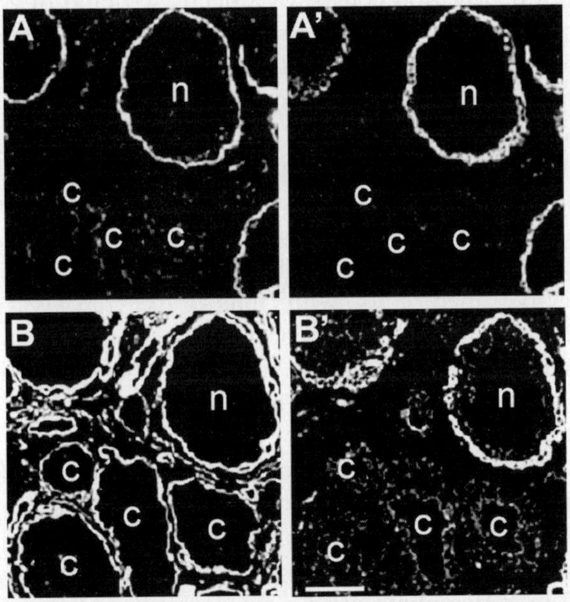

Figure 2. Immunofluorescence doublestaining of prostate serial sections (A,B) with laminin 5 (A) and cytokeratin 5 (A') and with laminin 10 (B) and cytokeratin 5 (B'). Normal prostate glands (n) express laminin 5, laminin 10 and cytokeratin 5, while cancer glands (c) express laminin 10, but no laminin 5 and no cytokeratin 5. Bar, 30 μm.

4. PROSTATIC STEM CELLS

In contrast to other epithelial tissues, such as the epidermis and the gut, there is little information about stem cells in the prostate. It has been proposed that (located within the basal cell layer), the prostate contains a small stem cell population that gives rise to a more rapidly amplifying cell population, which then differentiates into the luminal secretory cells and into neuroendocrine cells (5,10,30,38). Evidence for the existence of prostate stem cells comes from castration studies. Androgens are required for normal prostate development as well as for maintenance and function of the organ in the adult (39). Following castration, the androgen deprived adult prostate undergoes rapid atrophy with loss of up to 90 % of the total epithelial cells, predominantly luminal secretory cells, via apoptosis (39, 40). The cells that remain are androgen-independent. However, some of these cells are androgen responsive, since the regressed prostate retains the ability to completely regenerate following restimulation with androgens (39). Presumably, a reservoir of androgen receptive stem cells accounts for the regeneration of the prostate. Interestingly, there is marked decrease in the prevalence and extent of high grade PIN following androgen deprivation therapy when compared to untreated cases (41). The morphological changes during androgen deprivation consist of a decreased ratio of acini to stroma, glandular atrophy, cytoplasmic clearing with increased apoptosis (42). The role of androgen hormones in prostate cancer is essentially permissive, because androgens are required for normal glandular homeostasis (43, 44). Although androgen receptor (AR) gene amplification may influence androgen sensitivity of prostatic glandular epithelial cells, AR gene mutations have been reported in only a minority of prostate carcinomas. The AR gene is polymorphic demonstrating variable lengths of CAG repeats in different men. Prostate epithelial cells with short CAG repeats are more androgen sensitive then cells with long CAG repeats (43). African-Americans carry the shortest CAG repeats, Caucasians have an intermediate length, and Asians have the longest. Correspondingly, the incidence and mortality of prostate cancer is highest in African-Americans. The lowest risk is seen in Asians.

At present, the identification of stem cells is complicated by the lack of unique structural markers. Cell division cannot be used as an indication of stem cell status. Cell kinetic studies indicate that stem cells are usually quiescent or slow dividing and that most of the dividing cells in the tissue are committed to differentiate after a finite number of divisions, but they possess a high proliferation potential (45). Stem cells need to overcome the loss of telomeres which is necessary for unlimited division. Usually, most somatic tissues express undetectable levels of telomerase. Normal adult rat prostate glands are telomerase negative, whereas residual glands of long-term castrates enriched in stem cells express high levels of telomerase (46). In normal human prostate tissue, the luminal cells are found to be negative and the basal cells positive for the human telomerase (hTR) mRNA (46). In addition, pp32 expression, a nuclear phosphoprotein, has been shown by *in situ* hybridization to be restricted to the basal cells of normal human prostate and was proposed as a candidate for a prostate stem cell marker (47). Prostate stem cell antigen, homologue to stem cell antigen 2 in the hematopoietic development, has also been shown to be expressed on the cell surface in a subset of prostate basal cells (48). Because of its cell surface expression it also has been proposed as a useful marker for the localization and especially the isolation of putative prostate stem cells (49). GSTP1, the pi class glutathione S-transferases catalyzing the conjugation of reduced glutathione to chemically reactive electrophiles and probably involved in the defense against organic hydroperoxides, has been reported to be predominantly expressed in the basal cells of normal prostate and to be absent from most prostatic adenocarcinomas (50). Low expressions of $p27^{Kip1}$, a member of the cip/kip family of cyclin dependent kinase inhibitors involved in cell cycle arrest, has been shown in proliferating cells (51). In normal prostate, most of the secretory cells are positive for $p27^{Kip1}$, however its expression in the basal cell layers is rather heterogeneous (49). P27Kip1-negative cells are considered to be highly proliferation competent (52).

More recently, studies examining the heterogeneity of prostate epithelial cells identified phenotypes which are intermediate between those of the basal and luminal layers expressing a mixture of basal and luminal markers such as cytokeratins (10, 36). These intermediate cell phenotypes are believed to represent the transit amplifying cell population. Another study showed that cytokeratin 19, which has been implicated in the differentiation of many different epithelial tissues in which there is a transition between differentiated phenotypes such as oral epithelium, mammary gland ducts, and the outer root sheath of the hair follicle, may be an useful marker for the amplifying non-stem-cell basal population in the prostate (53). All carcinomas express cytokeratin 8 and 18 and most, including PIN lesions, express cytokeratin 19 (36) and not cytokeratin 14. It is therefore possible that these tumors arise from a cytokeratin 14 negative/cytokeratin 19 positive cell population. Recently, human prostate epithelial cells with stem cell characteristics were isolated on the basis of rapid adhesion to type 1 collagen and the expression of higher levels of the $\alpha 2$ integrin subunit, which co-expressed CD 133 (54-56). These selected cells showed a basal phenotype by cytokeratin 5 and 14 expression and lacked PSA and PAP expression and showed a fourfold greater ability to form colonies *in vitro* than the total basal cell population (54). In the proximal regions of murine prostatic ducts a candidate population of prostatic stem cells was identified recently by high level expression of stem cell antigen 1 (Sca-1) in conjunction with α6 integrin and bcl-2 expression (57).

5. PROSTATE MORPHOGENESIS

Studies of the young adult prostate showed persistent foci and segments that retained a prepubertal appearance (4), which reflected perhaps earlier developmental differences in prostate tissue. This asynchronous postpubertal prostatic development was similar to the focal and regional asynchrony of development observed in fetal prostates (58). Moreover, in a mouse model of prostate carcinoma, developmental asynchrony was one of the characteristic observations (59). It has been postulated that these developmentally abnormal foci and segments of prostate predispose to prostatitis (60). Geographic differences in fetal development of the prostate corresponding with the geographic variations in clinical carcinogenesis, would suggest re-conceptualizing the pathogenesis of adult prostate disease (58, 59). Maternal hormonal influences might account for the observed developmental differences. This process, referred to as neonatal imprinting or developmental estrogenization, is associated with an increased incidence of prostatic lesions upon aging, which include hyperplasia, inflammation and dysplasia similar to PIN (61, 62). It is hypothesized that these molecular and cellular changes initiated early in life predispose the prostate to the neoplastic state upon aging.

Prostatic development, which is androgen-dependent, is initiated prenatally but is not completed until the end of puberty. Androgen production by the developing fetal testis begins (week 8 in human) before and continues throughout periods of prostatic morphogenesis (63). While testosterone is the primary androgen produced by the fetal testis, dihydrotestosterone (DHT) appears to be responsible for prostatic morphogenesis. DHT is produced within the endodermal urogenital sinus (UGS) by enzymatic reduction of testosterone by 5-α-reductase, which has been detected in the UGS of humans and rodents (63). The concentrations of androgens are relatively high at the end of gestation, decrease one day after birth, remain low until puberty, and increase to adult concentrations (64). The prostatic ductal networks are derived from solid epithelial outgrowth (prostatic buds) that emerge from the UGS below the developing bladder and grow into the surrounding mesenchyme. The normal human prostatic ductal morphogenesis and growth occur in two separate periods, prenatally and pubertally (63). In the human fetus, the prostate begins to form around the 10th week of gestation (65, 66). By 13 weeks of gestation there are approximately 70 primary ducts, some of which exhibit secretory cyto-differentiation (65, 66). At about 34 weeks' gestation, acinotubular structures appear in the more peripheral zone.

The epithelial cells of the prostatic buds co-express cytokeratins 5, 8, 14 and 18, and p63 (67). As the solid epithelial cords canalize from the urethral terminus towards the ductal tips, the epithelium differentiate into two distinct cell populations, luminal and basal cells expressing their characteristic subset of cytokeratins. At the same time, the prostatic mesenchyme/stroma differentiates into a layer of smooth muscle that surrounds the prostatic ducts (68).

In contrast to the mouse prostate, some secretory activity was found to be detectable during fetal life in the human prostate (58). Multiple paracrine signaling events between the developing prostatic mesenchyme and epithelium are required both for normal branching morphogenesis and for the differentiation of specialized stromal and epithelial cell types (63). Recently, some genes required for prostate development were identified. These included several transcription factors including the androgen receptor (69), and three homeodomain-containing transcription factors Hox-a13, Hox-d13 (70, 71), and Nkx3.1 (72). The following growth factors have been implicated in the regulation of prostate development and adult tissue homeostasis: the fibroblast growth factors FGF7 (also known as keratinocyte growth factor, KGF) and FGF10 (73, 74), the insulin-like growth factor 1 (75), TGF-β (76), and sonic hedgehog (77). The latter was shown to activate mesenchymal Gli1 expression, a member of the Gli gene family of transcriptional regulators, during prostate ductal bud formation (78). Furthermore, α-(1,2) fucosyl-transferase and H-type 2 carbohydrate structures were implicated as important mediators of prostatic development (79). In addition, the tyrosine kinase colony-stimulating factor-1 receptor (CSF-1R) was found to be correlated with murine prostatic development, proliferation and cancer progression (80). p63 -/- mice were shown not to develop a recognizable prostate (81). CD 44, a marker of early progenitor cells within the prostatic epithelium, was shown to be expressed by actively proliferating epithelia at sites of epithelial-mesenchymal interaction (82). Hyaluronan (HA), the extracellular ligand of CD 44, was shown to be highly expressed in the proliferating distal buds of the developing ducts in the developing prostate (83). This suggested a significant role of hyaluronan-CD 44 interactions in mediating androgen-induced prostatic growth and morphogenesis. Recently, another study showed that the disruption of urokinase plasminogen (uPA) binding to the uPA receptor resulted in a retardation of the development of the ventral prostrate in newborn rats (83).

The bone morphogenetic protein 4 (Bmp4), a member of the TGF-β superfamily was shown to inhibit prostatic ductal branching (84). The secreted factors activin A and its binding protein follistatin have been implicated in regulating prostate morphogenesis (85). Activin A was shown to inhibit prostatic branching morphogenesis, and follistatin was shown to increase branching *in vitro* (85).

In spite of this progress, these genes do not completely explain the complex molecular mechanism behind the regulation of prostatic development.

6. CYTOKERATIN 6 EXPRESSION IN PROSTATE STEM CELLS

Recently, we discovered in human prostate tissue a new epithelial cell phenotype with stem cell properties that expresses cytokeratin 6 as observed by RT-PCR (Figure 3), Western blotting, immunofluorescence microscopy, and immunohistochemistry (86).

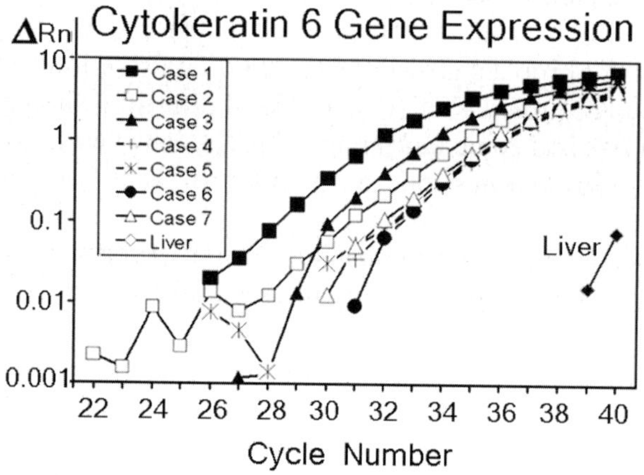

Figure 3. Normal, non-cancerous areas of the prostates of 7 patients were analyzed for cytokeratin 6 gene expression by RT-PCR. The primers were targeted to the 3rd and 5th exons of cytokeratin 6 gene (accession numbers ay 033496, ay 033495). Human liver was used as negative control.

The types of cytokeratins that are expressed, constituting intermediate filaments in epithelial tissue, is closely linked to the differentiation state of the epithelium. Cytokeratin 6 is constitutively expressed in certain complex epithelial such as the foot sole and the inner differentiating layer of the outer root sheath of the hair follicle, but are absent from the interfollicular epidermis (87). Cytokeratin 6 was reported to be implicated with hyperproliferation and aberrant differentiation such as psoriasis and cancer and to be up-regulated in keratinocytes at the wound edge in skin (87). The cytokeratin 6 positive cells (ck6+ cells) exhibited the following stem cell properties: (1) a niche like distribution pattern; (2) a proliferation potential; (3) a differential potential; (4) the presence of cytokeratin 6 positive cells in fetal, juvenile and adult prostate glands; (5) cytokeratin 6 positive cells were abundant in the urogenital sinus known to be enriched in stem cells.

(1) In adult normal human prostate tissue, the cytokeratin 6 expressing cells occurred in the basal cell compartment within specialized niches (Figure 4) that are consistent with stem cell niches and co-expressed cytokeratin 5.

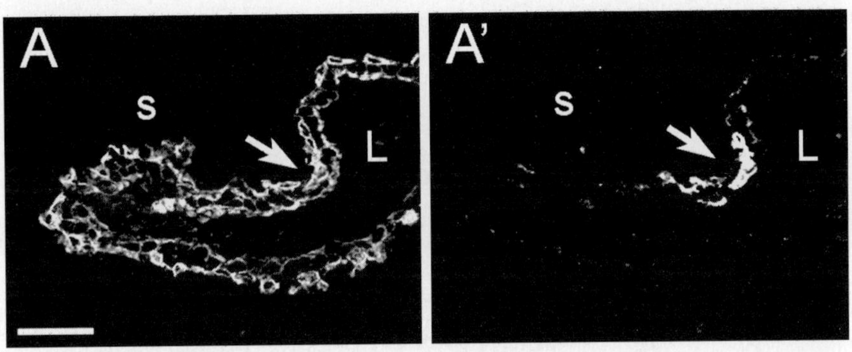

Figure 4. Immunofluorescence doublestaining of cytokeratin 5 (A) and cytokeratin 6 (A') in a normal human prostate gland. (A) and (A') show the same field of view in the same section. S, stroma, L, lumen. The arrow points to the stem cell niche-like distribution pattern within the basal cell layer. Bar, 20 μm.

The average abundance of ck6+ cells was 4.9% in the adult slow cycling normal prostate with a proliferation rate of 1.1%.

(2) Recently a "Prostate Organ Culture Model" was described in which tissue cores obtained from prostatectomies were sliced into ~ 250 nm thick slices (88). These tissue slices then were cultured up to 5 days with intact

epithelial-stromal interaction. In this model, the presence of growth factor enriched serum stimulated cytokeratin 5 positive basal cells to proliferate as well as migrate from cut open glands to the surface to form and cover the stroma with a new surface epithelium. The coring of the prostate gland specimen for tissue slice acquisition for this *in vitro* study model led to wounding of prostatic glands and stroma, a tissue damage to which a stem cell and the resulting transient amplifying cells would be expected to respond. Consistent with such a stem cell response, the number of cytokeratin 6 expressing cells increased to 64.9% in this prostate organ culture model with co-expression of cytokeratin 5. The proliferation rate increased to 5.84% with 98.76 % of all proliferating cells being cytokeratin 6 positive. In this tissue model, the increase of ck6+ cells significantly correlated with the increased proliferation rate (Pearson's correlation coefficient $r = 0.7616$, $p = 0.0467$).

(3) Classically defined stem cells have a capacity to generate daughter cells that can differentiate into several cell lineages to form all the cell types that constitute the mature epithelium (88). Consistent with this concept, we demonstrated that ck6+ cells were able to differentiate into luminal cells in the normal adult prostate gland (Figure 5) and to form a newly differentiated surface epithelium in the prostate organ culture model.

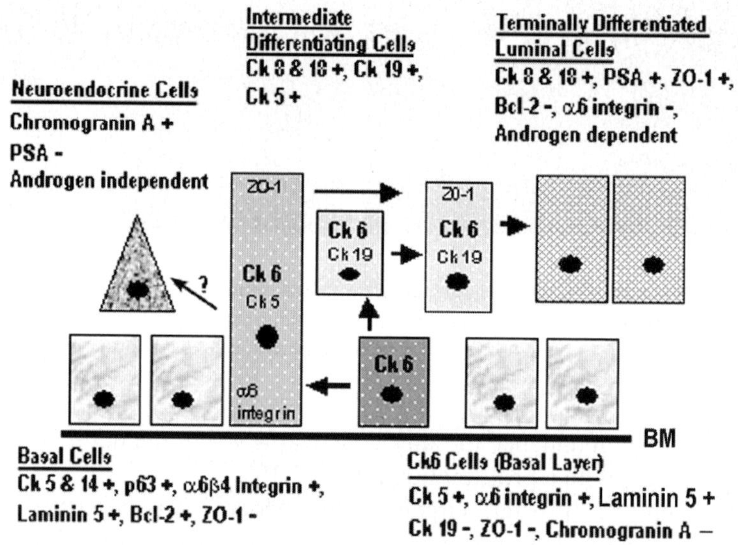

Figure 5. Schematic of the distribution and protein expression pattern of cytokeratin 6 positive cells in the normal adult human prostate epithelium. BM, basement membrane.

When migrating from the basal layer to the luminal layer in the adult prostate epithelium ck6+ cells co-expressed cytokeratin 19 or ZO-1 (Figures 5, 6). Cytokeratin 19, which has been implicated in the differentiation of many epithelial tissues in which there is a transition between different phenotypes (90), was shown to be a marker for prostatic intermediate cells and to play a key role in prostatic differentiation (91).
ZO-1, a tight junctional protein, is exclusively expressed by terminally differentiated luminal cells, but not by basal cells in the normal adult prostate (Figure 6).

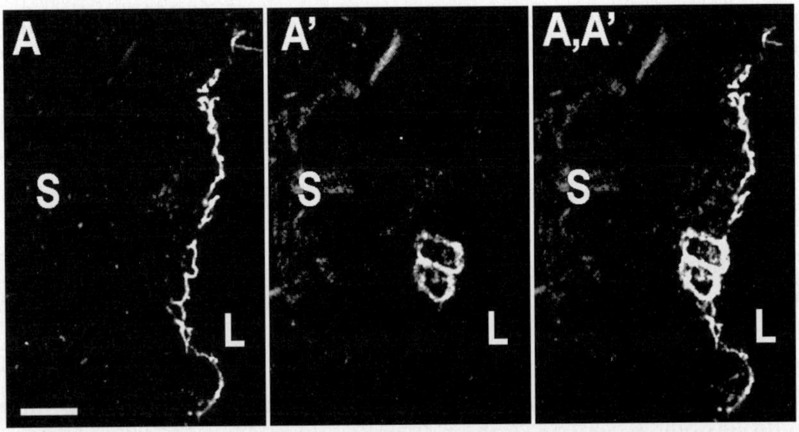

Figure 6. Immunofluorescence doublestaining of the tight junctional protein ZO-1 (A) with cytokeratin 6 (A') in normal adult human prostate, (A,A') shows the overlay of (A) and (A'). Note that cytokeratin 6 cells in the luminal compartment co-express ZO-1. Bar, 10 µm, S, stroma, L, glandular lumen.

This suggests that the ck6+ cells that co-express ZO-1 are transient amplifying cells that are committed for terminal differentiation, and which later may lose cytokeratin 6 expression. The newly formed surface epithelium of the prostate organ culture model expressed cytokeratin 6, and formed ultrastucturally a new basement membrane with deposition of the extracellular matrix proteins laminin 5 and collagen VII, and also showed differentiation into basal and luminal cells as demonstrated by conventional electron microscopy and PSA expression (86). This further indicated that cytokeratin 6 expression may be maintained beyond the stem cell stage.

(4) In the juvenile prostate (age 9 months to 12 years) and in the fetal prostate (22–39 weeks of gestation) cytokeratin 6 was expressed focally in

single cells or in cell clusters in both the basal and luminal cells showing a similar expression pattern as in the adult normal prostate. In the fetal prostate, in addition to cytokeratin 6 expression in the glandular epithelium, isolated cytokeratin 6 positive cells were located in the mesenchymal stroma both adjacent and distant to glands. In the actively proliferating epithelia of the developing human fetal prostate, a remarkable number of ck+ 6 cells was proliferative co-expressing Ki-67.

(5) Cytokeratin 6 was also abundantly expressed in the urogenital sinus, which gives rise to the urinary bladder and to the prostate and is enriched in stem cells, and in the developing bladder as shown by immunohistochemistry.

In summary, our data suggest a major role of the ck6+ cells in prostate morphogenesis.

7. THE IMPORTANCE OF UNDERSTANDING PROSTATE MORPHOGENESIS

The composition of normal prostatic epithelium includes the complex interaction of the phenotypically distinct cell types. It has now become apparent how these individual cell lineages share a common origin, and are related in a precursor-progeny sequence. In this precursor-progeny sequence the basal epithelial compartment plays a fundamental role in normal prostatic growth as well as in the initiation and progression of at least some forms of prostate cancer. Because prostate disease, both malignant and benign, involves inappropriate cell division and differentiation, it is important to identify the stem cell and amplifying populations, and to understand the role of different cell phenotypes, especially the role of the ck6+ cells, in the maintenance of tissue homeostasis and development of the prostatic tissue. Stem cells are considered the major targets of oncogenesis. A large replicative potential and a long life enables stem cells to accumulate multiple mutations over time, which makes them likely candidates for the cells of origin of cancer. The knowledge of the features of the prostatic stem cells could help to understand the mechanism involved in prostatic carcinogenesis. Ductal morphogenesis is common to normal developing prostate, BPH, and prostatic adenocarcinoma. All forms of prostatic growth, normal and neoplastic, exhibit androgen dependency at least initially. Since it is unlikely that different biological mechanisms would be utilized to produce prostatic ductal architecture in all three growth states, the developmental biology of the prostate provides a potentially important model for understanding proliferative diseases of the prostate gland.

ACKNOWLEDGEMENT

The authors would like to thank Dr. Bernard W. Futscher at the Arizona Cancer Center (University of Arizona, Tucson, AZ) for his expert help with the cytokeratin 6 gene expression (RT-PCR) experiments. This work was supported in part by the US Department of Veterans Affairs (VISN18 grant 2004) and by DOD Award W81XWH-04-1-0921.

REFERENCES

1. American Cancer Society: Cancer Facts and Figures. Atlanta, GA. American Cancer Society, 2004.
2. Ekman, P. Genetic and environmental factors in prostate cancer genesis: identifying high-risk cohorts. Eur Urol. 35(5-6):362-9, 1999.
3. Gardner, W. Hypothesis: the prenatal origins of prostate cancer. Human Pathology 26: 1291-1292, 1995.
4. Gardner, W., Culberson, D. Atrophy and proliferation in the young adult prostate. J Urol. 137: 53-56, 1987.
5. Isaacs, J., Coffey, D. Etiology and disease process of benign prostatic hyperplasia. The Prostate 2: 33-50, 1989.
6. Reya, T., Morrison S., Clarke, M., Weissman, I. Stem cells, cancer and cancer stem cells. Nature 414: 105-111, 2001.
7. di, Sant'Agnese, P., Cockett, A. Neuroendocrine differentiation in prostatic malignancy.Cancer 78: 357-361, 1996.
8. Liu, A, True, L., LaTray, L., Nelson, P., Ellis, W., Vessella, R., Lange, P., Hood, L., Van den, Engh, G. Cell-cell interaction in prostate gene regulation and cytodifferentiation. Proc Nat Acad Sci, USA 94: 10705-10710, 1997.
9. McDonnell, T., Troncoso, P., Brisbay, S., Logothetis, C., Chung, L., Hsieh, J., Tu, S., Campbell, M. Expression of the protooncogene bcl-2 in the prostate and its association with emergence of androgen-independent prostate cancer. Cancer Res. 52: 6940-6944, 1992.
10. Bonkhoff, H., Stein, U., Remberger, K. Multidirectional differentiation in the normal, hyperplastic, and neoplastic human prostate. Hum Pathol. 25: 42-46, 1994.
11. Sherwood, E., Berg, L., Mitchell, N., McNeal, J., Kozlowski, J., Lee, C. Differential cytokeratin expression in normal hyperplastic and malignant epithelial cells from human prostate. J Urol. 143:167-171, 1990.
12. Nagle, R., Hao, J., Knox, J., Dalkin, B., Clark, V., Cress, A. Expression of hemidesmosomal and extracellular matrix proteins by normal and malignant human prostate tissue. Am J Pathol. 146: 1498-507, 1995.

13. Brar, P.K., Dalkin, B.L., Weyer, C., Sallam, K., Virtanen, I., Nagle, RB. Laminin alpha-1, alpha-3, and alpha-5 chain expression in human prepubetal benign prostate glands and adult benign and malignant prostate glands. The Prostate, 55 (1): 65-70, 2003.
14. Bissell, M., Nelson, W. Cell-to-cell contact and extracellular matrix. Integration of form and function: the central role of adhesion molecules. Curr Opin Cell Biol. 11: 537, 1999.
15. Green, K., Jones, J. Desmosomes and hemidesmosomes: Structure and function of molecular components. FASEB J. 10: 871-880, 1996.
16. Olumi, A.F., Grossfeld, G.D., Hayward, S.W., Carroll, P.R., Tlsty, T.D., Cunha, G.R. Carcinoma-associated Fibroblasts Direct Tumor Progression of Initiated Human Prostatic Epithelium. Cancer Res. 59: 5002-5011, 1999.
17. Sakr, W.A., Haas, G.P., Cassin, B.J., Pontes, J.E., Crissman, J.D. Frequency of carcinoma and intraepithelial neoplasia of the prostate in young male patients. J. Urol 150: 379-385; 1993.
18. Sakr, W.A., Grignon, D.J., Crissman, J.D., Heilbrun, L.K., Cassin, B.J., Pontes, J.J., Haas, G.P. High grade prostatic intraepithelial neoplasia (HGPIN) and prostatic adenocarcinoma between the ages of 20-69. An autopsy study of 249 cases. In Vivo 8: 439-443; 1994.
19. Qian, J., Wollan, P., Bostwick, D.G. The extent and multicentricity of high grade prostatic intraepithelial neoplasia in clinically localized prostatic adenocarcinoma. Hum Pathol 28 (2): 143-148, 1997.
20. Bostwick, D.G. Target populations and strategies for chemoprevention trials of prostate cancer. J Cell Biochem Suppl.19:191-6, 1994.
21. Sakr, W.A., Grigon, D.J., Haas, G.P., Schomer, K.L., Heilbrun, L.K., Cassin, B.J., Powerll, I.J., Montie, J.A., Pontes, J.E., Crissman, J.D. Epidemiology of high grade prostatic intraepithelial neoplasia. Pathol Res Pract 19 (9): 838-41, 1995.
22. Bostwick, D.G., Qian, J., Frankel, K. The incidence of high grade prostatic intraepithelial neoplasia in needle biopsies. J Urol. 154 (5):1791-4, 1995.
23. DeMarzo, A.M., Nelson, W.G., Isaacs, W.B., Epstein, J.I. Pathological and molecular aspects of prostate cancer. Lancet 361(9361):955-64, 2003.
24. Montironi, R., Galluzzi, C.M., Diamanti, L., Giannulus, I., Pisani, E., Scarpelli, M. Prostatic intra-epithelial neoplasia: expression and location of proliferating cell nuclear antigen in epithelial, endothelial and stromal nuclei. Virchows Arch A Pathol Anat Histopathol. 422(3):185-92, 1993.
25. Isaacs, J.T. Molecular markers of prostate cancer metastasis. Am J Pathol 150: 1511, 1997.
26. Lara, P.N. Jr., Kung, H.J., Gumerlock, P.H., Meyers, F.J. Molecular biology of prostate carcinogenesis. Crit Rev Oncol Hematol. 32 (3): 197-208, 1999.
27. Ruijter, E., Montironi, R., van de Kaa, C., Schalken, J. Molecular changes associated with prostate cancer development. Anal Quant Cytol Histol 23 (1):67-88, 2001.
28. Cress, A.E., Rabinovitz, I., Zhu, W., Nagle, R.B. The $\alpha6\beta1$ and $\alpha6\beta4$ integrins in human prostate cancer progression. Cancer Metastasis Rev 14: 219-228, 1995.
29. Schmelz, M., Cress, A.E., Scott, K.M., Bürger, F., Cui, H., Sallam, K., McDaniel, K.M., Dalkin, B.L., Nagle, R.B. Different Phenotypes in Human Prostate Cancer : $\alpha6$ or $\alpha3$ Integrin in Cell-Extracellular Adhesion Sites. Neoplasia 4 (3), 2002.
30. Bonkhoff, H., Remberger, K. Differentiation pathways and histogenetic aspects of normal and abnormal prostatic growth: a stem cell model. The Prostate 28: 98-106, 1996.
31. Bussemakers, M., van Bokhoven, A., Tomita, K., Jansen, C.F., Schalken, J.A. Complex cadherin expression in human prostate cancer cells. Int J Cancer 85: 446-450, 2000.

32. Zha, S., Ferdinandusse, S., Denis, S., Wanders, R.J., Ewing, C.M., Luo, J., De Marzo A.M., Isaacs, WB. Alpha-methylacyl-CoA racemase as an androgen-independent growth modifier in prostate cancer. Cancer Res: 63 (21): 7365-76, 2003.
33. Rhodes, D.R., Sanda, M.G., Otte, A.P., Chinnaiyan, A.M, Rubin, M.A. Multiplex biomarker approach for determining risk of prostate specific antigen defined recurrence of prostate cancer. J Natl Cancer Inst. 95: 66-81, 2003.
34. Cheng, L., Song, S.Y., Pretlow, T.G., Abdul-Karim, F.W., Kung, H.J., Dawson, D.V., Park, WS, Moon, Y.W., Tsai, M.L., Linehan, W.M., Emmert-Buck, M.R., Liotta, L.A., Zhuang, Z. Evidence of independent origin of multiple tumors from patients with prostate cancer. J Natl. Cancer Inst. 90: 233-7, 1998.
35. Wheeler, T.M., Rogers, E., Aihara, M., Scardino, P.T., Thompson, T.C. Apoptotic index as a biomarker in prostatic intraepithelial neoplasia (PIN) and prostate cancer. J Cell Biochem 19: 202-7, 1994.
36. Verhagen, A.P., Ramaekers, F.C., Aalders, T.W., Schaafsma, H.E., Debruyne, F.M., Schalken, J.A. Colocalization of basal and luminal cell-type cytokeratins in human prostate cancer. Cancer Res 52: 6182, 1992.
37. Djakiew, D. Dysregulated expression of growth factors and their receptors in the development of prostate cancer. The Prostate 42: 150-160, 2000.
38. Bui, M., Reiter, R. Stem cell genes in androgen-independent prostate cancer. Cancer and Metastasis Reviews 17: 391-399, 1999.
39. Hayward, S., Baskin, L., Haughney, P., Cunha, A., Foster, B., Dahiya, R., Prins, G., Cunha, GR. Epithelial development in the rat ventral prostate, anterior prostate and seminal vesicle. Acta Anat (Basel) 155: 81-93, 1996.
40. English, H., Santen, R., Isaacs, J. Response of glandular versus basal rat ventral prostatic epithelial cells to androgen withdrawal and replacement. The Prostate 11: 229-42, 1987.
41. Ferguson, J., Zincke, H., Ellison, E., Bergstrahl, E., Bostwick, D.G. Decrease of prostatic intraepithelial neoplasia (PIN) following androgen deprivation therapy in patients with stage T3 carcinoma treated by radical prostatectomy. Urol 44:91-95, 1994.
42. Trapman, J., Brinkman, A.O. The androgen receptor in prostate cancer. Patho Res Prect 192: 752-60, 1996.
43. Nelson, W.G., De Marzo, A.M., Isaacs, W.B. Prostate cancer. New Engl. J Med. 349: 366, 2003.
44. Gronberg, H. Prostate cancer epidemiology. Lancet 361: 859, 2003.
45. Potten, C., Loeffler, M. Stem cells: attritubes, cycles, spirals, pitfalls and uncertainties. Lessons for and from the crypt. Development 110: 1001-20, 1990.
46. Paradis, V., Dargere, D., Laurendeau, I., Benoit, G., Vidaud, M., Jardin, A., Bedossa, P. Expression of the RNA component of human telomerase (htr) in prostate cancer, prostatic intraepithelial neoplasia, and normal prostate tissue. J Pathol. 189: 213-218, 1999.
47. Walensky, L., Coffey, D., Chen, T., Wu, T., Pasternack, G. A novel M(r) 32,000 nuclear phosphoprotein is selectively expressed in cells competent for self-renewal. Cancer Res. 53: 4720-6, 1993.
48. Reiter, R., Gu, Z., Watabe, T., Thomas, G., Szigeti, K., Davis, E., Wahl, M., Nisitani, S., Yamashiro, J., Le Beau, M., Loda, M., Witte, O. Prostate stem cell antigen: a cell surface marker overexpressed in prostate cancer. Proc Natl Acad Sci USA. 95: 1735, 1998.
49. De Marzo, A., Nelson, W., Meeker, A., Coffey, D. Stem cell features of benign and malignant prostate epithelial cells. J Urol. 160: 2381-2392, 1998.

50. Moskaluk, C., Duray, P., Cowan, K., Linehan, M., Merino, M. Immunohistochemical expression of pi-class glutathione S-transferase is down-regulated in adenocarcinoma of the prostate. Cancer 79: 1595, 1997.
51. Sherr, C. Cancer cell cycles. Science 274: 1675, 1996.
52. De Marzo, A., Meeker, A., Epstein, J., Coffey, D. Prostate stem cell compartments: expression of p27Kip1 in normal, hyperplastic and cancer cells. American Journal of Pathology 153: 911-918, 1998.
53. Hudson, D.L., Guy, A.T., Fry, P., O'Hare, M.J., Watt, F.M., Master, JRW. Epithelial Cell Differentiation Pathways in the Human Prostate: Identification of Intermediate Phenotypes by Keratin Expression. J. Histochem. Cytochem. 49: 271-278, 2001.
54. Collins, A., Habib, F., Maitland, N., Neal, D. Identification and isolation of human prostate epithelial stem cells based on $\alpha 2\beta 1$-integrin expression. Journal of Cell Science 114: 3865-3872, 2001.
55. Hudson, D., O'Hare, M., Watt, F., Masters, J. Proliferative heterogeneity in the human prostate: evidence for epithelial stem cells. Laboratory Investigations 80: 1243-1250, 2000.
56. Richardson, G.D., Robson, C.N., Lang, S.H., Neal, D.E., Maitland, N.J., Collins, A.T. CD 133, a novel marker for human prostatic stem cells. J Cell Sci 117: 3539-3545, 2003.
57. Burger, P.E., Xiong, X., Coetzee, S., Salm, S.N., Moscatelli, D., Goto, K., Wilson, E.L. Sca-1 expression identifies stem cells in the proximal region of prostatic ducts with high capacity to reconstitute prostatic tissue. PNAS, 102 (20): 7180-7185, 2005.
58. Xia, T., Blackburn, W., Gardner, W. Fetal prostate growth and development. Pediatr Pathol. 10: 527-537, 1990.
59. Sugimura, Y., Sakurai, M., Hayashi, N., Yamashita, A., Kawamura, J. Age-related changes of the prostate gland in the senescence-accelerated mouse. The Prostate 24: 24-32, 1994.
60. Gardner, W., Bennett, B. The prostate-overview: recent insights and speculations. In Gardner, W.A., Weinstein, R.S. (eds): Pathology and Pathobiology of Urinary Bladder and Prostate. Baltimore, Williams & Wilkins. 129-148, 1992.
61. Pylkkanen, L., Makela, S., Valve, E., Harkonen, P., Toikkanen, S., Santti, R. Prostatic dysplasia associated with increased expression of C-MYC in neonatally estrogenized mice. J. Urol. 149: 1593-601, 1993.
62. Prins, G. Developmental estrogenization of the prostate gland. In: Prostate: Basic and Clinical Aspects. (Ed. R.K. Naz, CRC Press: Boca Raton, FL). 247-65, 1997.
63. Cunha, G., Donjacour, A., Cooke, P., Mee, S., Bigsby, R., Higgins, SJ., Sugimura, Y. The endocrinology and developmental biology of the prostate. Endocrine Reviews 8:338-362, 1987.
64. Thomson, A. Role of androgens and fibroblast growth factors in prostatic development. Reproduction 121: 187-195, 2001.
65. Lowsley, O. The development of the human prostate gland with reference to the development of other structures at the neck of the urinary bladder. Am J Anat. 13: 299, 1912.
66. Kellokumpu-Lethinen, P., Santti, R., Pelliniemi, L. Correlation of early cyto-differentiation of the human fetal prostate and Leydig cells. Anat. Rec. 196: 263, 1980.
67. Wang, Y., Hayward, S., Cao, M., Thayer, K., Cunha, GR. Cell differentiation lineage in the prostate. Differentiation 68: 270-279, 2001.
68. Hayward, S., Baskin, L., Haughney, P., Foster, B., Cunha, A., Dahiya, R., Prins, G., Cunha, G.R. Epithelial development in the rat ventral prostate, anterior prostate and seminal vesicle. Acta Anat (Basel)155: 81-93, 1996.

69. Donjacour, A., Cunha, G.R. Assessment of prostatic protein secretion in tissue recombinants made of urogenital sinus mesenchyme and urothelium from normal or androgen-insensitive mice. Endocrinology 131: 2342-2350, 1993.
70. Podlasek, C., Clemens, J., Bushman, W. Hoxa-13 gene mutation results in abnormal seminal vesicle and prostate development. J. Urol. 161: 1655-1661, 1999.
71. Oefelein, M., Chin-Chance, C., Bushman, W. Expression of the homeotic gene Hox-d13 in the developing and adult mouse prostate. J. Urol. 155: 342-346, 1996.
72. Bhatia-Gaur, R., Donjacour, A.A, Sciavolino, P.J., Kim, M., Desai, N., Young, Norton C.R., Gridley, T., Cardiff, R.D., Cunha, G.R., Abate-Shen, C., Shen, M.M. Roles for Nkx3.1 in prostatedevelopment and cancer. Genes Dev. 13: 966-977, 1999. Acta Anat (Basel) 155: 94-103,1996.
73. Sugimura, Y., Foster, B., Hom, Y., Lipschutz, J., Rubin, J., Finch, P., Aaronson, S., Hayashi, N. Kawamura, J., Cunha, G.R. Keratinocyte growth factor (KGF) can replace testosterone in the ductal branching morphogenesis of the rat ventral prostate. Int. J. Dev. Biol. 40: 941-951, 1996.
74. Thomson, A., Cunha, G.R. Prostatic growth and development are regulated by FGF10. Development 126: 3693-3701, 1999.
75. Ruan, W., Powell-Braxton, L., Kopchick, J., Kleinberg, D. Evidence that insulin-like growth factor 1 and growth hormone are required for prostate gland development. Endocrinology 140: 1984-1989, 1999.
76. Salm, S.N., Burger, P., Coetzee, S., Goto, K., Moscatelli, D., Wilson, E.L. TGF-β maintains dormancy of prostatic stem cells in the proximal region of ducts.
77. Wang, B.-E., Shou, J., Ross, S., Koeppen, H., de Sauvage, F.J., Gao, W.-Q. Inhibition of Epithelial Ductal Branching in the Prostate by Sonic Hedgehog Is Indirectly Mediated by Stromal Cells. J. Biol. Chem. 278: 18506-18513, 2003.
78. Lamm, M., Catbagan, W., Laciak, R., Barnett, D., Hebner, C., Gaffield, W., Walterhouse, D., Iannaccone, P. Sonic hedgehog activates mesenchymal Gli1 expression during prostate ductal bud formation. Developmental Biol. 249: 349-366, 2002.
79. Marker, P., Stephan, J.P., Lee, J., Bald, Mather J., Cunha, G.R. Fucosyltransferase 1 and H-Type complex carbohydrates modulate epithelial cell proliferation during prostatic branching morphogenesis. Dev. Biol. 233: 95-108, 2001.
80. Ide, H., Seligson, D., Memarzadeh, S., Xin, L., Horvath, S., Dubey, P., Flick, M., Kacinski, B., Palotie, A., Witte, O. Expression of colony-stimulating factor 1 receptor during prostate development and prostate cancer progression. PNAS 99: 14404-14409, 2002.
81. Signoretti, S., Waltregny, D., Dilks, J., Isaac, B., Lin, D., Garraway, L., Yang, A., Montironi, R., McKeon, F., Loda, M. p63 Is a Prostate Basal Cell Marker and Is Required for Prostate. Development. Am J Pathol. 157: 1769-1775, 2000.
82. Gakunga, P., Frost, G., Shuster, S., Cunha, G., Formby, B., Stern, R. Hyaluronan is a prerequisit for ductal branching morphogenesis. Development 124: 3987-3997, 1997.
83. Elfman, F., Bok, R., Conn, M., Shuman, M., Cunha, G.R. Urokinase plasminogen activator amino-terminal peptides inhibit development of the rat ventral prostate. Differentiation 69: 108-120, 2001.
84. Lamm, M., Podlasek, C., Barnett, D., Lee, J., Clemens, J., Hebner, C., Bushman, W. Mesenchymal factor bone morphogenetic protein 4 restricts ductal budding and branching morphogenesis in the developing prostate. Developmental Biol. 232: 301-314, 2001.

85. Cancilla, B., Jarred, R., Wang, H., Mellor, S., Cunha, G., Risbridger, G. Regulation of prostate branching morphogenesis by activin A and follistatin. Dev. Biol. 237: 145-158, 2001.
86. Schmelz, M., Moll, R., Hesse, U., Prasad, A.R., Gandolfi, J.A., Hasan, S.R., Bartholdi, M., Cress, A.E. Identification of a stem cell candidate in the normal human prostate gland. Eur J Cell Biol 84: 341-354.
87. McGowan, K., Coulombe, P. The wound repair-associated keratins 6, 16 and 17. Insights into the role of intermediate filaments in specifying keratinocyte cytoarchitecture. Subcellular Biochemistry: Intermediate Filaments, eds. Herrmann and Harris. 31: 173-204, 1998.
88. Parrish, A., Sallam, K., Nyman, D., Orozco, J., Cress, A.E., Dalkin, B., Nagle, R., Gandolfi, A. Culturing precision-cut human prostate slices as an in vitro model of prostate pathobiology. Cell Biol Toxicol 18: 205-219, 2002.
89. Smalley, M., Ashworth, A. Stem cells and breast cancer: a field in transit. Nat Rev Cancer 3: 832-844, 2003.
90. Stasiak, P., Purkis, P., Leigh, I., Lane, E. Keratin 19: predicted amino acid sequence and broad tissue distribution suggest it evolved from keratinocyte keratins. J Invest Dermatol 92: 707-716, 1989.
91. Hudson, D.L., Guy, A., Fry, P., O'Hare, M.J., Watt, F.M., Masters, J.R.W. Epithelial Cel Differentiation pathways in the human prostate : Identification of intermediate phenotypes by keratin expression. J Histochem Cytochem 49: 271-278, 2001.

Chapter 7

EPIGENETIC REGULATION OF GENES THAT AFFECT TUMOR CELL ADHESION

Bernard W. Futscher[1] and Frederick E. Domann[2]
[1]*Department of Pharmacology and Toxicology, College of Pharmacy, Arizona Cancer Center, University of Arizona, Tucson, AZ, USA;.* [2]*Free Radical and Radiation Biology Program, Department of Radiation Oncology, Carver College of Medicine and Holden Cancer Center, University of Iowa, Iowa City, IA, USA*

Abstract: During cancer progression there is an accumulation of genetic and epigenetic changes that dictate the phenotypic diversity of a tumor population. Epigenetics is a heritable change in phenotype that is independent of a change in the genotype. The focus of this chapter is to review, in part, the literature indicating that an "epigenetic switch" occurs in cancer progression and to detail the evidence of one particular gene product, maspin, as a paradigm of epigenetic control. The regulation of maspin expression in normal epithelial tissue and the multiple mechanisms by which maspin is inappropriately silenced in cancer is discussed. Understanding the molecular features of the epigenetic switch is likely to provide a therapeutic opportunity to induce transcriptional reprogramming and prevent devastating disease processes such as epithelial cancer metastasis.

Key words: maspin; epigenetics; epithelial cancer; CpG islands; DNA methylation; Histone deacetylation; breast cancer; prostate cancer

1. INTRODUCTION

Cancer progression is characterized by the acquisition of genetic and epigenetic changes that lead to generation of phenotypic diversity among the progeny of cancer cells. The evolution of this diversity allows for the continual selection of cells that possess the most suitable attributes for

A.E. Cress and R.B. Nagle (eds.), Cell Adhesion and Cytoskeletal Molecules in Metastasis, 123–140.

survival under any given set of conditions in the host. As the cancer cells undergo their dispersion, it is likely that critical, but potentially transient changes in gene expression programs occur as cancer cells break away from a primary tumor and invade local tissues and metastasize to distant sites. One gene that may promote survival in one physiological context (e.g., primary tumor site, metastatic colony site) may be deleterious in another physiological context (invasive disseminating tumor). For this reason, epigenetic alterations in gene expression patterns could account for loss of gene expression under one set of circumstances yet allow for the re-expression of this gene should its function provide a selective advantage later in cancer progression.

Similar to genetic instability, epigenetic instability is also a hallmark of malignant cells (1, 2). Unlike the permanent genetic alterations of mutation, translocation and deletion, epigenetic changes are metastable and can be reversed in tumor cells and normal cells. As such, if a cell adopts a new gene expression pattern as a result of epigenetic alterations or perturbation, that cell and its progeny retain the capability to switch back to previous gene expression patterns. This phenotypic plasticity provides unstable cancer cells the ability to change their gene expression programs and suitably adapt to the various environment encountered during the trip from primary lesion to metastatic colony. We suggest that cancer cells can modulate the expression of genes involved in cell adhesion and motility or the transcription factors that control their expression during cancer progression. These genes may remain active in the primary tumor during early cancer development; however, as natural selection occurs these genes need be silenced so that the tumor has the necessary phenotypic characteristics for malignant transformation. Following cancer cell colonization at a distant site, the malignant tumor may require reacquisition of those gene products that suppress the properties of motility and invasion. Regulation of the expression of this complement of genes, through epigenetic mechanisms, provides a switch mechanism in tumor cells that is not as drastic as mutation, and is readily reversible. In support of this possibility, some tumor suppressor genes, such as p53, are typically mutated and deleted, and rarely, if ever, are silenced in association with DNA methylation (3). In contrast, some genes with tumor suppressor function, rarely, if ever, are mutated, and often are silenced by aberrant DNA methylation. Examples of this latter class of genes include MGMT, maspin, GST pi, desmocollin 3 and 14-3-3 sigma (4-11).

2. THE EPIGENETIC MARK

One critical epigenetic mark found on the DNA is 5-methylcytosine. In mammalian cells, 5-methylcytosine occurs exclusively in the nucleotide doublet, 5'-CpG-3', and is the only modified base found in the human genome that is not recognized as DNA damage. It is estimated that 60 – 80% of the CpG cytosines are methylated in the human genome. In the human genome very high levels of 5-methylcytosine exist in high copy repetitive elements such as alpha satellite sequences that comprise pericentromeric heterochromatin, most ALU elements, as well as many single copy regions of the genome. The regions of the genome where unmethylated CpGs concentrate are genomic elements termed CpG islands (12).

CpG islands comprise about 1% of the genome, are on average 1kb in length, and are interesting because they typically are found overlapping the transcription start site of all housekeeping genes and perhaps 50% of tissue-restricted genes (13). The unmethylated state of CpG islands keeps the region in an "open" or accessible topological conformation, and renders the region transcriptionally competent, but not necessarily transcriptionally active (14, 15). In addition, there are regions of the genome that display cell type specific patterns of DNA methylation and these cell type specific patterns can be seen from the level of the whole chromosome down to the level of the individual gene. Importantly these DNA methylation differences are associated with differences in expression of the affected genes (9, 16-24).

It appears that in all cancers the normal patterns of 5-methylcytosine are disrupted resulting in both known and unknown consequences. The earliest work on cancer cells demonstrated a genome-wide hypomethylation (25-28). Much of this loss of methylation can be found to recur consistently in satellite sequences; although the functional consequences of these changes in DNA methylation have not yet been fully elucidated, it is likely that they serve an important function in the transformed phenotype. Additionally, it has been speculated that demethylation may also activate oncogenes by allowing for their overexpression or inappropriate expression, although incontrovertible evidence remains lacking.

Aberrant methylation or hypermethylation of specific DNA sequences is also detected in human tumor cells, even in the face of overall genomic hypomethylation (29). CpG island promoters represent an important target of aberrant or inappropriate methylation, and this aberrant methylation is intimately linked with the transcriptional silencing of the associated gene (30). Targets for aberrant methylation in cancer include cell cycle regulatory genes, genes involved in maintenance of genomic integrity, and metastasis suppressor genes that encode cell adhesion molecules and motility factors.

With respect to gene regulatory sequences, it is well documented that hypermethylation of CpG island regulatory sequences results in the silencing of tumor suppressor genes (5, 7, 8, 29, 31-36). Interestingly, the patterns of aberrant methylation of CpG islands have been shown to be tumor type tumor type specific (4).

A number of epigenetic marks exist along with 5-methylcytosine, and it appears that these marks act in concert to control genome structure and function. As such, epigenetic regulation is a multifaceted control system, in which 5-methylcytosine is just one of many aspects. Another critical facet of epigenetic regulation is post translational modifications to the histones around which the DNA is wrapped. The most compelling evidence indicates that the histone modifications work in concert with 5-methylcytosine to repress transcriptional activity of associated genomic regions. 5-methylcytosine can recruit proteins to the genomic region it is localized, and these proteins can act as transcriptional repressors and proceed to alter the DNA topology of the region to render it transcriptionally inactive – the region no longer is readily accessible for binding by the transcription machinery. One of the more completely delineated aspects of this epigenetic regulation has demonstrated that densely methylated DNA recruits methylcytosine binding proteins to the region, which in turn recruits histone deacetylase complexes that deacetylate histones H3 and H4; a change in the histone modification state that is associated with gene silencing, whereas acetylation of multiple lysine residues on histones H3 and H4 is associated with a transcriptionally competent or active state (37-40). Other histone modifications are also critical in controlling the epigenetic state (e.g., histone methylation), and the interplay of these histone modifications with each other and with DNA methylation is an area of intense research activity (41-43). The control of these epigenetic changes and their temporal relationship remain an enigmatic and controversial area.

3. MASPIN

The gene Maspin (SERPBINB5) represents a paradigm for the study of epigenetic dysregulation of genes that are involved in cell invasion and metastasis. Maspin expression in normal tissue is controlled, in part, by epigenetic mechanisms and this underlying mechanism is compromised in cancer leading to the inappropriate silencing of maspin in cancers derived from maspin-positive cell types, as well as the activation of maspin in cancers derived from normally maspin-negative cell types. During malignant transformation, epigenetic instability and mischief results in a loss of control in the expression of many genes that are similar to maspin with respect to the malignant phenotype. We propose that these genes, through metastable epigenetic switching mechanisms, can be turned off and on in response to environmental stresses and cues in the cancer cell, thereby allowing tumor cells a phenotypic plasticity that appears necessary for the challenges a tumor cell and its progeny must undertake to migrate from primary tumor site to distant metastatic site.

Maspin (derived from **mam**mary ser**pin**) was one of the first tumor suppressor genes isolated using expression genetics, and is based on the idea that investigation of heredity at the level of RNA and gene expression would reveal many new genes and pathways involved in oncogenesis (44). Using the techniques of subtractive hybridization and differential display, Ruth Sager and her laboratory used this approach to discover genes down-regulated at the level of gene transcription that was not due to gene mutation or deletion (45). Maspin is a significant example of the genes found by the Sager laboratory approach.

The original publication emanating from the Sager laboratory reported the results of a functional genomics screen used to identify genes down-regulated in breast cancer when compared to normal breast cells grown under similar conditions (46). More than 30 such genes were identified with one of the genes isolated being maspin. The cell biology studies described in the original report clearly showed that maspin has tumor suppressor function in breast cancer and are discussed briefly below. Human breast cancer cells transfected with a maspin cDNA showed a reduction in the number and size of tumors that formed in the mouse mammary fat pad xenograft model. Reintroduction of maspin also blocked the malignant potential of the tumors that did form in the mouse xenografts, evidenced by the fact that no metastases were found in the lymph nodes or lungs of maspin transfected breast cancer cells. Surprisingly, compared to the *in vivo* effects of maspin reintroduction, no difference in growth rates between maspin transfectants and controls were seen *in vitro* cell culture, suggesting that the inhibitory effect on tumor formation and dissemination was not a result of a simple maspin-induced growth inhibition. Functional analysis of maspin's effects *in vitro* revealed that the maspin transfectants have a diminished invasive potential compared to control cells. Immunohistochemical analysis of human breast cancers for maspin protein expression indicated that maspin was lost in a high percentage of lymph node metastases and pleural effusions. Taken together, the results presented in this study implicate strongly a critical role for the loss of maspin expression in the evolution of human breast cancer.

In the initial report, Southern blot analysis showed that the maspin gene was present and not grossly rearranged or mutated in breast cancer cells where maspin expression was lost. Additionally, treatment of cells with the tumor promoter TPA was able to re-induce maspin gene expression. It is tempting to speculate that many of the other genes that the Sager laboratory isolated using this paradigm may very well be inappropriately silenced by the same mechanisms responsible for silencing maspin gene expression.

4. MASPIN GENETICS AND EPIGENETICS

The maspin gene is located at chromosome 18.q21.33 and consists of seven exons stretching across a region of about 30kb, with the first exon being non-coding. Three maspin gene mRNA transcripts have been detected with the major transcript that produces the mature protein being approximately 3kb in size as assessed by northern blot analysis. The two other transcripts arising from the maspin gene are of unknown function (and are not always detectable). One transcript is approximately 1.2 kb and shares extensive homology with the 5' end of the maspin gene, and the other transcript being approximately 4.6 kb that appears to be an incomplete splice variant of maspin (http://genome.ucsc.edu/).

In normal human cells, maspin expression is limited largely to epithelial cell types, such as breast, prostate, skin, oral, and bronchial epithelial cells, although exceptions exist, such as corneal stromal cells (47). In contrast, maspin is not expressed in most non-epithelial cell types, such as peripheral blood mononuclear cells, cardiac muscle, fibroblasts, chondrocytes. Because maspin expression is regulated primarily at the level of transcription, and is frequently lost or down-regulated in cancer, detailed analysis of the maspin promoter should provide meaningful insights into the mechanism of gene control and aberrant silencing of maspin in breast cancer.

The earliest studies on the maspin promoter emanated, not surprisingly, from the Sager laboratory. Studies in breast and prostate cancer cells, using deletion and mutation constructs of the maspin promoter in chloramphenicol acetyltransferase reporter assays and electromobility shift assays, provided the first data regarding transcription factors important to basal maspin expression (48, 49). These studies clearly demonstrated the importance of the AP-1 and its transcription factors in the positive regulation of maspin in breast and prostate tissue, and set the stage for all subsequent work regarding the control of maspin transcription. Exciting recent work identified p53 binding sites in the maspin promoter region (50). These investigators demonstrated that introduction of wild-type p53 could activate maspin expression in prostate cancer cells as well as the p53 wild-type breast cancer cell line, MCF7. Our laboratories' followed up these observations with microarray-based studies in which we examined p53 target genes (34). The analysis of the resultant gene expression using multidimensional scaling supported the hypothesis that maspin is a p53-inducible gene. In this study we also demonstrated direct binding of p53 to the maspin promoter using *in vivo* chromatin immunoprecipitation assays. Finally, a pair of studies published in the past few months provides the intriguing observation, that the p53 homolog p63, which can bind the same recognition sequence as p53, can substitute for p53 and induce maspin gene expression when expressed in cancer cells (51, 52). The important role of p63 in development and differentiation of epithelial cell types including epidermis, mammary, prostate – all maspin positive cell types – suggests the intriguing possibility that cell type specific maspin expression is established at least in part through p63 dependent mechanism during development.

Further analysis of this region indicated that the maspin promoter area fits the criteria of a CpG island original described by Frommer and Gardiner-Garden (13). In addition, other features, such as the fact that this region overlaps the promoter and transcriptional start site supports the CpG "islandness" of the region. Based on our interest in epigenetic control, this is where the story gets a little more interesting.

Analysis of the patterns of CpG methylation in the maspin promoter of normal cell types derived from a variety of different tissues revealed striking differences in CpG methylation that were tightly linked to the expression state of maspin and the overall chromatin structure of the region (9). Normal maspin-positive cell types (e.g. mammary, prostate, skin epithelium) have a uniformly unmethylated maspin promoter, the associated histones H3 and H4 are hyperacetylated, the K9 position of histone H3 is unmethylated, and the chromatin is in an accessible conformation. In contrast, maspin-negative tissue (e.g. lymphocytes, fibroblasts, chondrocytes) have a completely methylated maspin promoter, which is linked to hypoacetylated histones H3 and H4, methylation of K9 in histone H3, and an inaccessible chromatin structure (9) and unpublished results). Furthermore treatment of immortalized maspin-negative cells (such as the fibroblast strain VA-13) with the inhibitor of DNA methylation, 5-aza 2'deoxycytidine, led to a dose-dependent activation in maspin expression. These results provide evidence for a definitive role for CpG methylation in the establishment and maintenance of cell type specific gene expression, and provide support to the hypothesis proposed more than 25 years ago, that CpG methylation participates in the cell-type specific control of gene expression (53, 54).

The remainder of this chapter will briefly discuss the biologic role of the maspin protein, in an effort to emphasize the potential multifaceted roles and therefore importance of maspin in human cancer, especially breast cancer. The majority of discussion will be reserved for the control of maspin gene expression in normal tissue and the multiple mechanisms by which maspin may be inappropriately silenced (or activated) in normal and cancerous human tissue.

5. MASPIN EPIGENETICS AND CANCER

We reproduced and extended Sager's results in showing that maspin expression is lost in a high percentage of breast cancer cells (7). In an attempt to better understand the mechanism of the inappropriate silencing, we followed the Sager paradigm that the silencing was not genetic, but epigenetic in nature. We used bisulfite sequencing to analyze DNA methylation patterns and levels in breast cancer cells, and discovered that silencing of the maspin gene was frequently associated with aberrant methylation of the maspin promoter. In addition, we showed that this aberrant CpG methylation was associated with an inaccessible chromatin structure, through the use of nuclease sensitivity assays. Relief of this transcriptionally inactive state should allow for re-expression of maspin by allowing the transcription factors present to access their cognate binding sites within the maspin promoter. Treatment of a different breast cancer cell lines with the DNA methylation inhibitor 5-aza 2'-deoxycytidine was capable of reactivating maspin expression; strongly suggesting that at least one facet of the defect in maspin expression is epigenetic in nature. This initial *in vitro* observation has been confirmed and extended by a variety of other groups. More recent examination of the epigenetic state of the maspin promoter shows that histones associated with the maspin promoter become hypoacetylated in breast cancer (6, 34), as well as enriched for K9 methylation of histone H3 (unpublished observations). Table 1 contains our analysis of the epigenetic state of the maspin promoter in a set of different human breast cancer cell lines.

An important question to answer was whether aberrant methylation of the maspin promoter occurred in breast cancer *in vivo*. The cell type specific nature of maspin promoter methylation makes the analysis of methylation changes in tumor tissue challenging; only purified cell populations will lead to a definitive answer. We conducted a study of maspin expression and methylation state of 30 Ductal Carcinoma In-Situ (DCIS) specimens and two healthy controls using immunohistochemical analysis, laser capture microdissection, and bisulfite sequencing (55). Results also showed that 57% of the DCIS lost maspin expression; and for those for which sufficient amounts of genomic DNA could be isolated by laser capture microdissection, we found loss of maspin immunoreactivity was frequently, but not always, accompanied by aberrant methylation of the maspin promoter. Additionally, we found that the DCIS samples themselves often

Table 1. Epigenetic State of Maspin in Human Breast Cancer Cell Lines

Cell line	Maspin Expression	Promoter Methylation	Histone Acetylation H3	Histone Acetylation H4	Chromatin State
HMEC	++++	-	+	+	OPEN
MCF10	++++	-	+	+	OPEN
UACC 245	++	-			
ZR-71	+	-			
MCF7	-	+	-	-	CLOSED
BT549	-	+	-	-	
HS578T	-	+			
MDA-MB-435	-	+	-	-	CLOSED
MDA-MB-231	-	+	-	-	CLOSED
MDA-MB-157	-	+			
MDA-MB-453	-	+			
UACC 1179	-	+	-	-	CLOSED
UACC 893	-	+			
UACC 3133	-	+			
UACC 2087	-	-			
MDA-MB-468	-	-			

Maspin expression was determined by quantitative real time PCR using TaqMan chemistry. Maspin promoter methylation state was determined by sodium bisulfite sequencing. The histone aceylation state of the Maspin promoter was determined by chromatin immunoprecipitation assays using real time PCR with TaqMan chemistry. Chromatin structure was determined using a nuclease sensitivity assay coupled to linker-mediated PCR.

displayed significant heterogeneity in maspin staining within the tumor population, while normal tissue stained uniformly throughout the duct with intense staining in myoepithelial cells, consistent with earlier studies (56, 57). These results indicate that maspin silencing can be an early event in breast carcinogenesis and precede metastatic growth. Additionally, these studies also suggest that other mechanisms, in addition to CpG methylation, participate and perhaps cooperate with aberrant methylation to inappropriately silence maspin expression early in breast carcinogenesis.

Changes in maspin expression in cancer have been widely reported since its original identification in breast cancer. Many of these reports provide further support for the association of maspin gene expression changes with epigenetic changes, with both silencing due to aberrant hypermethylation and activation due to aberrant hypomethylation. Table 2 shows the human cancers where differences in maspin expression have been found between the tumor and the corresponding normal cell type, and if these differences in expression have been experimentally associated with the DNA methylation state.

Table 2. Human Cancer, Maspin Expression and the Epigenetic State

Tumor Type	Maspin Expression	Maspin Promoter Methylation	References
Breast	Silenced	Hypermethylation	(6, 7, 34, 55, 58, 59)
Prostate	Decreased	No Change	(59-63)
Pancreas	Activated	Hypomethylation	(64-68)
Thyroid	Activated	Hypomethylation	(19,69)
Ovarian	Activated	Hypomethylation	(70) and unpublished results
Lung	Activated	Hypomethylation	(51, 71-73)
Gastric	Conflicting	Hypomethylation	(74-78)
Melanoma	Activated	Hypomethylation	(79)
Oral	Decreased	Unknown	(80 ,81)
Salivary	Variable	Unknown	(82)
Bladder	Silenced	Unknown	(83, 84)
Colon	Variable	Unknown	(85, 86)

Maspin expression and promoter methylation status for each tumor type were taken from the references provided in the last column. Expression, in this case, refers to either mRNA or protein expression. DNA methylation state was provided if the referenced studies asayed CpG methylation status directly.

The loss of maspin expression seen in some tumors is confounded by the activation of maspin expression seen in other tumors. These apparently conflicting results have caused some concern regarding maspin's tumor suppressor role. A few points; however, should be made regarding the observations of maspin activation in cancer. The seemingly paradoxical activation of maspin in some tumors was described in correlative clinical studies where a role for maspin in the disease process has not been ascertained. One possibility for these surprising results is that the maspin protein has different functions in different cell types that is dependent on the spectrum of other maspin interacting proteins present within a given cell type and environment. Secondly, complex epigenetic changes occur to the genomes of cancer cells, and we have shown that the cell type specific expression of maspin is controlled by the cytosine methylation state of its promoter. As epigenetic modifications by their nature are metastable, it is possible that as the tumor evolves, a variety of epigenetic states emerge, and those which are most favorable to the current microenvironment conditions will likely be selected for and survive. Alternatively, epigenetic changes maybe neutral or unfavorable to tumor growth and dissemination. In this scenario, the activation of maspin in tumor cells derived from normal cells in a tissue that does not express maspin (e.g., pancreas) may be a result of complex epigenomic changes in DNA methylation. It is unknown if inappropriate activation of maspin expression imparts any significant phenotypic changes on the tumor at particular stages of cancer progression or whether its activation is an epiphenomenon that reflects loss of methylation homeostasis.

From these apparently conflicting results, it is clear additional studies will be required to unravel the complex question of how maspin expression may modify the malignant phenotype in some cell types and potentially not others. Nevertheless, it is clear the CpG methylation state plays an important role in in controlling maspin expression in normal tissue, and that this epigenetic control is compromised during human carcinogenesis.

6. MASPIN AS A PARADIGM OF EPIGENETIC CONTROL OF CELL TYPE SPECIFIC GENE EXPRESSION

Maspin is a clear example of an autosomal gene controlled by epigenetic mechanisms in normal healthy human tissue. Normal epithelial cells that are maspin-positive invariably have an unmethylated maspin promoter that is associated with heavily acetylated histones H3 and H4. These epigenetic marks are tightly linked to a chromatin structure that renders the promoter available for interaction with the transcriptional machinery. In contrast, normal human cell types that are derived from maspin-negative mesenchymal tissues uniformly have a methylated maspin promoter that is associated with underacetylated histones H3 and H4 and a closed chromatin structure that is blocks access to the transcriptional machinery.

Maspin gene expression is lost through epigenetic silencing in breast cancer. The epigenetic state of the maspin promoter in breast cancer cells closely resembles the epigenetic state of normal mesenchymal tissues that maintain maspin in a silent and inaccessible state. The breast cancer cells acquire a repressive chromatin structure through aberrant methylation of the promoter, deacetylation of the associated histones H3 and H4, as well as methylation of K9 residue of histone H3. Conversely, it is also noted that tumors derived from maspin-negative cell types often activate maspin gene expression, which is accompanied by demethylation of the maspin promoter and hyperacetylation of histones H3 and H4.

In cancer cells that undergo metastatic dispersal, we suggest that critical, but potentially transient, changes in gene expression patterns occur in an epigenetically-driven fashion. A gene that may promote survival in one physiological context (e.g., primary tumor site) may be deleterious in another context (e.g., invasive disseminating tumor), and vice versa. We propose that epigenetic regulation through CpG methylation and histone modification provides a mechanism by which cell type-specific genes can be turned on and off without direct mutation to the gene itself. For this reason we feel that alterations in gene expression programs at "the flip of an epigenetic switch" would allow for adaptation of cancer cells to their environment is an appealing and viable possibility. In other words, epigenetic control of genes is unique because it is reversible, and thereby can confer a high degree of plasticity to the malignant phenotype.

If this prediction is correct, then other cell-type specific genes controlled by epigenetic mechanisms must also be present. As such, candidate genes as well as epigenomic screening approaches can be used for the discovery of such genes. A candidate gene approach has already identified MCJ, and others such as HoxA5 and 14-3-3 sigma have been speculated (87, 88). Indeed, we have recently found that the 14-3-3 sigma CpG island is virtually identical to the epigenetic landscape we found for maspin in epithelial and mesenchymal cell types (29).

7. SUMMARY

Unlike the genetic mutations that accumulate in a cancer cell, epigenetic marks can be reversed. Thus, when a cell adopts a new gene expression profile as a result of epigenetic change, that cell and its progeny retain the capability to revert back to a previous gene expression pattern. As such, with respect to the epigenetic state neoplastic progression could perhaps not be considered a long straight march toward an increasingly aggressive phenotype, but rather as a stochastic trial and error saunter toward an increasingly malignant phenotype in a "two steps forward, one step backward" manner. Importantly, CpG methylation and associated epigenetic modifications appear to be causally involved in gene silencing since pharmacological inhibitors of DNA methylation and histone modification can re-activate expression (6, 89-91). The ability to reverse these cancer-related changes in epigenetic control provides a therapeutic opportunity to target the epigenetic machinery and induce transcriptional reprogramming.

ACKNOWLEDGEMENTS

This work was supported by Public Health Service grants CA65662 to BWF and CA73612 to FED. The authors would like to thank the various people from the Futscher and Domann labs that have contributed to this research. They are Nick Holtan, Dr. Marc Oshiro, Dr. George Watts, Ryan Wozniak, Damian Junk, Jose Munoz-Rodriguez, and Matthew Fitzgerald, Dr. Hong Duan, Christin Hanigan, Dr. Yuanhui Huang, and Dr. Stephen Rose.

REFERENCES

1. Jones, P.A. and Baylin, S.B. The fundamental role of epigenetic events in cancer. Nat Rev Genet, 3: 415-428, 2002.
2. Jaenisch, R. and Bird, A. Epigenetic regulation of gene expression: how the genome integrates intrinsic and environmental signals. Nat Genet, 33 Suppl: 245-254, 2003.
3. Soussi, T. and Beroud, C. Assessing TP53 status in human tumours to evaluate clinical outcome. Nat Rev Cancer, 1: 233-240, 2001.
4. Costello, J.F., Fruhwald, M.C., Smiraglia, D.J., Rush, L.J., Robertson, G.P., Gao, X., Wright, F.A., Feramisco, J.D., Peltomaki, P., Lang, J.C., Schuller, D.E., Yu, L., Bloomfield, C.D., Caligiuri, M.A., Yates, A., Nishikawa, R., Su Huang, H., Petrelli, N. J., Zhang, X., O'Dorisio, M.S., Held, W.A., Cavenee, W.K., and Plass, C. Aberrant CpG-island methylation has non-random and tumour-type-specific patterns. Nat Genet, 24: 132-138, 2000.
5. Millar, D.S., Ow, K.K., Paul, C.L., Russell, P.J., Molloy, P.L., and Clark, S.J. Detailed methylation analysis of the glutathione S-transferase pi (GSTP1) gene in prostate cancer. Oncogene, 18: 1313-1324, 1999.
6. Maass, N., Biallek, M., Rosel, F., Schem, C., Ohike, N., Zhang, M., Jonat, W., and Nagasaki, K. Hypermethylation and histone deacetylation lead to silencing of the maspin gene in human breast cancer. Biochem Biophys Res Commun, 297: 125-128, 2002.
7. Domann, F.E., Rice, J.C., Hendrix, M.J., and Futscher, B.W. Epigenetic silencing of maspin gene expression in human breast cancers. Int J Cancer, 85: 805-810, 2000.
8. Esteller, M., Hamilton, S.R., Burger, P.C., Baylin, S.B., and Herman, J.G. Inactivation of the DNA repair gene O6-methylguanine-DNA methyltransferase by promoter hypermethylation is a common event in primary human neoplasia. Cancer Res, 59: 793-797, 1999.
9. Futscher, B.W., Oshiro, M.M., Wozniak, R.J., Holtan, N., Hanigan, C.L., Duan, H., and Domann, F.E. Role for DNA methylation in the control of cell type specific maspin expression. Nat Genet, 31: 175-179, 2002.
10. Lee, W.H., Morton, R.A., Epstein, J.I., Brooks, J.D., Campbell, P.A., Bova, G.S., Hsieh, W.S., Isaacs, W.B., and Nelson, W.G. Cytidine methylation of regulatory sequences near the pi-class glutathione S-transferase gene accompanies human prostatic carcinogenesis. Proc Natl Acad Sci U S A, 91: 11733-11737, 1994.
11. Oshiro, M.M., Futscher, B.W., Lisberg, A., Wozniak, R.J., Klimecki, W.T., Domann, F.E., and Cress, A.E. Epigenetic regulation of the cell type-specific gene 14-3-3sigma. Neoplasia, 7: 799-808, 2005.

12. Baylin, S.B., Herman, J.G., Graff, J.R., Vertino, P.M., and Issa, J.P. Alterations in DNA methylation: a fundamental aspect of neoplasia. Adv Cancer Res, 72: 141-196, 1998.
13. Gardiner-Garden, M. and Frommer, M. CpG islands in vertebrate genomes. J Mol Biol, 196: 261-282, 1987.
14. Bird, A.P. CpG-rich islands and the function of DNA methylation. Nature, 321: 209-213, 1986.
15. Bird, A.P., Taggart, M.H., Nicholls, R.D., and Higgs, D.R. Non-methylated CpG-rich islands at the human alpha-globin locus: implications for evolution of the alpha-globin pseudogene. Embo J, 6: 999-1004, 1987.
16. Li, E., Beard, C., and Jaenisch, R. Role for DNA methylation in genomic imprinting. Nature, 366: 362-365, 1993.
17. Lindsay, S., Monk, M., Holliday, R., Huschtscha, L., Davies, K.E., Riggs, A.D., and Flavell, R.A. Differences in methylation on the active and inactive human X chromosomes. Ann Hum Genet, 49 (Pt 2): 115-127, 1985.
18. Mohandas, T., Sparkes, R.S., and Shapiro, L.J. Reactivation of an inactive human X chromosome: evidence for X inactivation by DNA methylation. Science, 211: 393-396, 1981.
19. Ogasawara, S., Maesawa, C., Yamamoto, M., Akiyama, Y., Wada, K., Fujisawa, K., Higuchi, T., Tomisawa, Y., Sato, N., Endo, S., Saito, K., and Masuda, T. Disruption of cell-type-specific methylation at the Maspin gene promoter is frequently involved in undifferentiated thyroid cancers. Oncogene, 23: 1117-1124, 2004.
20. Schofield, P.N., Joyce, J.A., Lam, W.K., Grandjean, V., Ferguson-Smith, A., Reik, W., and Maher, E.R. Genomic imprinting and cancer; new paradigms in the genetics of neoplasia. Toxicol Lett, 120: 151-160, 2001.
21. Swain, J.L., Stewart, T.A., and Leder, P. Parental legacy determines methylation and expression of an autosomal transgene: a molecular mechanism for parental imprinting. Cell, 50: 719-727, 1987.
22. Venolia, L., Gartler, S.M., Wassman, E.R., Yen, P., Mohandas, T., and Shapiro, L.J. Transformation with DNA from 5-azacytidine-reactivated X chromosomes. Proc Natl Acad Sci U S A, 79: 2352-2354, 1982.
23. Zhang, Y., Shields, T., Crenshaw, T., Hao, Y., Moulton, T., and Tycko, B. Imprinting of human H19: allele-specific CpG methylation, loss of the active allele in Wilms tumor, and potential for somatic allele switching. Am J Hum Genet, 53: 113-124, 1993.
24. Feil, R., Walter, J., Allen, N.D., and Reik, W. Developmental control of allelic methylation in the imprinted mouse Igf2 and H19 genes. Development, 120: 2933-2943, 1994.
25. Feinberg, A.P. and Vogelstein, B. Hypomethylation distinguishes genes of some human cancers from their normal counterparts. Nature, 301: 89-92, 1983.
26. Feinberg, A.P. and Vogelstein, B. Alterations in DNA methylation in human colon neoplasia. Semin Surg Oncol, 3: 149-151, 1987.
27. Gama-Sosa, M.A., Slagel, V.A., Trewyn, R.W., Oxenhandler, R., Kuo, K.C., Gehrke, C.W., and Ehrlich, M. The 5-methylcytosine content of DNA from human tumors. Nucleic Acids Res, 11: 6883-6894, 1983.
28. Ehrlich, M. DNA methylation in cancer: too much, but also too little. Oncogene, 21: 5400-5413, 2002.
29. Baylin, S.B., Fearon, E.R., Vogelstein, B., de Bustros, A., Sharkis, S.J., Burke, P.J., Staal, S.P., and Nelkin, B.D. Hypermethylation of the 5' region of the calcitonin gene is a property of human lymphoid and acute myeloid malignancies. Blood, 70: 412-417, 1987.

30. Baylin, S.B. and Herman, J.G. DNA hypermethylation in tumorigenesis: epigenetics joins genetics. Trends Genet, 16: 168-174., 2000.
31. Graff, J.R., Herman, J.G., Lapidus, R.G., Chopra, H., Xu, R., Jarrard, D.F., Isaacs, W., Pitha, P.M., Davidson, N.E., and Baylin, S.B. E-cadherin expression is silenced by DNA hypermethylation in human breast and prostate carcinomas. Cancer Res, 55: 5195-5199, 1995.
32. Watts, G.S., Pieper, R.O., Costello, J.F., Peng, Y.M., Dalton, W.S., and Futscher, B.W. Methylation of discrete regions of the O6-methylguanine DNA methyltransferase (MGMT) CpG island is associated with heterochromatinization of the MGMT transcription start site and silencing of the gene. Mol Cell Biol, 17: 5612-5619, 1997.
33. Rice, J.C., Ozcelik, H., Maxeiner, P., Andrulis, I., and Futscher, B.W. Methylation of the BRCA1 promoter is associated with decreased BRCA1 mRNA levels in clinical breast cancer specimens. Carcinogenesis, 21: 1761-1765, 2000.
34. Oshiro, M.M., Watts, G.S., Wozniak, R.J., Junk, D.J., Munoz-Rodriguez, J.L., Domann, F.E., and Futscher, B.W. Mutant p53 and aberrant cytosine methylation cooperate to silence gene expression. Oncogene, 22: 3624-3634, 2003.
35. Merlo, A., Herman, J.G., Mao, L., Lee, D.J., Gabrielson, E., Burger, P.C., Baylin, S.B., and Sidransky, D. 5' CpG island methylation is associated with transcriptional silencing of the tumour suppressor p16/CDKN2/MTS1 in human cancers. Nat Med, 1: 686-692, 1995.
36. Herman, J.G., Merlo, A., Mao, L., Lapidus, R.G., Issa, J.P., Davidson, N.E., Sidransky, D., and Baylin, S.B. Inactivation of the CDKN2/p16/MTS1 gene is frequently associated with aberrant DNA methylation in all common human cancers. Cancer Res, 55: 4525-4530, 1995.
37. Wade, P.A., Gegonne, A., Jones, P.L., Ballestar, E., Aubry, F., and Wolffe, A.P. Mi-2 complex couples DNA methylation to chromatin remodelling and histone deacetylation. Nat Genet, 23: 62-66, 1999.
38. Meehan, R.R., Lewis, J.D., McKay, S., Kleiner, E.L., and Bird, A.P. Identification of a mammalian protein that binds specifically to DNA containing methylated CpGs. Cell, 58: 499-507, 1989.
39. Boyes, J. and Bird, A. DNA methylation inhibits transcription indirectly via a methyl-CpG binding protein. Cell, 64: 1123-1134, 1991.
40. Nan, X., Ng, H.H., Johnson, C.A., Laherty, C.D., Turner, B.M., Eisenman, R.N., and Bird, A. Transcriptional repression by the methyl-CpG-binding protein MeCP2 involves a histone deacetylase complex. Nature, 393: 386-389, 1998.
41. Strahl, B.D. and Allis, C.D. The language of covalent histone modifications. Nature, 403: 41-45, 2000.
42. Rea, S., Eisenhaber, F., O'Carroll, D., Strahl, B.D., Sun, Z.W., Schmid, M., Opravil, S., Mechtler, K., Ponting, C.P., Allis, C.D., and Jenuwein, T. Regulation of chromatin structure by site-specific histone H3 methyltransferases. Nature, 406: 593-599, 2000.
43. Lehnertz, B., Ueda, Y., Derijck, A.A., Braunschweig, U., Perez-Burgos, L., Kubicek, S., Chen, T., Li, E., Jenuwein, T., and Peters, A.H. Suv39h-mediated histone H3 lysine 9 methylation directs DNA methylation to major satellite repeats at pericentric heterochromatin. Curr Biol, 13: 1192-1200, 2003.
44. Pardee, A.B. Ruth Sager, Geneticist. In: M.J.C. Hendrix (ed.), Maspin, pp. 1-7. Georgetown: Landes Biosciences, 2002.
45. Zhang, M.S., S: Pardee, AB Maspin in the Sager Laboratory. In: M.J.C. Hendrix (ed.), Maspin. Georgetown: Landes Biosciences, 2002.

46. Zou, Z., Anisowicz, A., Hendrix, M.J., Thor, A., Neveu, M., Sheng, S., Rafidi, K., Seftor, E., and Sager, R. Maspin, a serpin with tumor-suppressing activity in human mammary epithelial cells. Science, 263: 526-529, 1994.
47. Ngamkitidechakul, C., Warejcka, D.J., Burke, J.M., O'Brien, W.J., and Twining, S.S. Sufficiency of the reactive site loop of maspin for induction of cell-matrix adhesion and inhibition of cell invasion. Conversion of ovalbumin to a maspin-like molecule. J Biol Chem, 278: 31796-31806, 2003.
48. Zhang, M., Maass, N., Magit, D., and Sager, R. Transactivation through Ets and Ap1 transcription sites determines the expression of the tumor-suppressing gene maspin. Cell Growth Differ, 8: 179-186, 1997.
49. Zhang, M., Magit, D., and Sager, R. Expression of maspin in prostate cells is regulated by a positive ets element and a negative hormonal responsive element site recognized by androgen receptor. Proc Natl Acad Sci U S A, 94: 5673-5678, 1997.
50. Zou, Z., Gao, C., Nagaich, A.K., Connell, T., Saito, S., Moul, J.W., Seth, P., Appella, E., and Srivastava, S. p53 regulates the expression of the tumor suppressor gene maspin. J Biol Chem, 275: 6051-6054, 2000.
51. Kim, S., Han, J., Kim, J., and Park, C. Maspin expression is transactivated by p63 and is critical for the modulation of lung cancer progression. Cancer Res, 64: 6900-6905, 2004.
52. Spiesbach, K., Tannapfel, A., Mossner, J., and Engeland, K. TAp63gamma can substitute for p53 in inducing expression of the maspin tumor suppressor. Int J Cancer, 114: 555-562, 2005.
53. Holliday, R. and Pugh, J.E. DNA modification mechanisms and gene activity during development. Science, 187: 226-232., 1975.
54. Riggs, A.D. X inactivation, differentiation, and DNA methylation. Cytogenet Cell Genet, 14: 9-25, 1975.
55. Futscher, B.W., O'Meara, M.M., Kim, C.J., Rennels, M.A., Lu, D., Gruman, L.M., Seftor, R.E., Hendrix, M.J., and Domann, F.E. Aberrant methylation of the maspin promoter is an early event in human breast cancer. Neoplasia, 6: 380-389, 2004.
56. Sternlicht, M.D., Safarians, S., Rivera, S.P., and Barsky, S.H. Characterizations of the extracellular matrix and proteinase inhibitor content of human myoepithelial tumors. Lab Invest, 74: 781-796, 1996.
57. Reis-Filho, J.S., Milanezi, F., Silva, P., and Schmitt, F.C. Maspin expression in myoepithelial tumors of the breast. Pathol Res Pract, 197: 817-821, 2001.
58. Maass, N., Hojo, T., Zhang, M., Sager, R., Jonat, W., and Nagasaki, K. Maspin--a novel protease inhibitor with tumor-suppressing activity in breast cancer. Acta Oncol, 39: 931-934, 2000.
59. Duan, H., Zhang, H.J., Yang, J.Q., Oberley, L.W., Futscher, B.W., and Domann, F.E. MnSOD up-regulates maspin tumor suppressor gene expression in human breast and prostate cancer cells. Antioxid Redox Signal, 5: 677-688, 2003.
60. Machtens, S., Serth, J., Bokemeyer, C., Bathke, W., Minssen, A., Kollmannsberger, C., Hartmann, J., Knuchel, R., Kondo, M., Jonas, U., and Kuczyk, M. Expression of the p53 and Maspin protein in primary prostate cancer: correlation with clinical features. Int J Cancer, 95: 337-342, 2001.
61. Zou, Z., Zhang, W., Young, D., Gleave, M.G., Rennie, P., Connell, T., Connelly, R., Moul, J., Srivastava, S., and Sesterhenn, I. Maspin expression profile in human prostate cancer (CaP) and in vitro induction of Maspin expression by androgen ablation. Clin Cancer Res, 8: 1172-1177, 2002.

62. Abraham, S., Zhang, W., Greenberg, N., and Zhang, M. Maspin functions as tumor suppressor by increasing cell adhesion to extracellular matrix in prostate tumor cells. J Urol, 169: 1157-1161, 2003.
63. Sheng, S., Carey, J., Seftor, E.A., Dias, L., Hendrix, M.J., and Sager, R. Maspin acts at the cell membrane to inhibit invasion and motility of mammary and prostatic cancer cells. Proc Natl Acad Sci U S A, 93: 11669-11674, 1996.
64. Ohike, N., Maass, N., Mundhenke, C., Biallek, M., Zhang, M., Jonat, W., Luttges, J., Morohoshi, T., Kloppel, G., and Nagasaki, K. Clinicopathological significance and molecular regulation of maspin expression in ductal adenocarcinoma of the pancreas. Cancer Lett, 199: 193-200, 2003.
65. Maass, N., Nagasaki, K., Ziebart, M., Mundhenke, C., and Jonat, W. Expression and regulation of tumor suppressor gene maspin in breast cancer. Clin Breast Cancer, 3: 281-287, 2002.
66. Maass, N., Hojo, T., Ueding, M., Luttges, J., Kloppel, G., Jonat, W., and Nagasaki, K. Expression of the tumor suppressor gene Maspin in human pancreatic cancers. Clin Cancer Res, 7: 812-817, 2001.
67. Sato, N., Fukushima, N., Matsubayashi, H., and Goggins, M. Identification of maspin and S100P as novel hypomethylation targets in pancreatic cancer using global gene expression profiling. Oncogene, 23: 1531-1538, 2004.
68. Fitzgerald, M., Oshiro, M., Holtan, N., Krager, K., Cullen, J.J., Futscher, B.W., and Domann, F.E. Human pancreatic carcinoma cells activate maspin expression through loss of epigenetic control. Neoplasia, 5: 427-436, 2003.
69. Ito, Y., Yoshida, H., Tomoda, C., Uruno, T., Takamura, Y., Miya, A., Kobayashi, K., Matsuzuka, F., Matsuura, N., Kuma, K., and Miyauchi, A. Maspin expression is directly associated with biological aggressiveness of thyroid carcinoma. Thyroid, 14: 13-18, 2004.
70. Sood, A.K., Fletcher, M.S., Gruman, L.M., Coffin, J.E., Jabbari, S., Khalkhali-Ellis, Z., Arbour, N., Seftor, E.A., and Hendrix, M.J. The paradoxical expression of maspin in ovarian carcinoma. Clin Cancer Res, 8: 2924-2932, 2002.
71. Heighway, J., Knapp, T., Boyce, L., Brennand, S., Field, J.K., Betticher, D.C., Ratschiller, D., Gugger, M., Donovan, M., Lasek, A., and Rickert, P. Expression profiling of primary non-small cell lung cancer for target identification. Oncogene, 21: 7749-7763, 2002.
72. Smith, S.L., Watson, S.G., Ratschiller, D., Gugger, M., Betticher, D.C., and Heighway, J. Maspin - the most commonly-expressed gene of the 18q21.3 serpin cluster in lung cancer - is strongly expressed in preneoplastic bronchial lesions. Oncogene, 22: 8677-8687, 2003.
73. Yatabe, Y., Mitsudomi, T., and Takahashi, T. Maspin expression in normal lung and non-small-cell lung cancers: cellular property-associated expression under the control of promoter DNA methylation. Oncogene, 23: 4041-4049, 2004.
74. Son, H.J., Sohn, T.S., Song, S.Y., Lee, J.H., and Rhee, J.C. Maspin expression in human gastric adenocarcinoma. Pathol Int, 52: 508-513, 2002.
75. Wang, M.C., Yang, Y.M., Li, X.H., Dong, F., and Li, Y. Maspin expression and its clinicopathological significance in tumorigenesis and progression of gastric cancer. World J Gastroenterol, 10: 634-637, 2004.
76. Zheng, H.C., Wang, M.C., Li, J.Y., Yang, X.F., Sun, J.M., and Xin, Y. Expression of maspin and kai1 and their clinicopathological significance in carcinogenesis and progression of gastric cancer. Chin Med Sci J, 19: 193-198, 2004.

77. Ito, R., Nakayama, H., Yoshida, K., Oda, N., and Yasui, W. Loss of maspin expression is associated with development and progression of gastric carcinoma with p53 abnormality. Oncol Rep, 12: 985-990, 2004.
78. Akiyama, Y., Maesawa, C., Ogasawara, S., Terashima, M., and Masuda, T. Cell-type-specific repression of the maspin gene is disrupted frequently by demethylation at the promoter region in gastric intestinal metaplasia and cancer cells. Am J Pathol, 163: 1911-1919, 2003.
79. Wada, K., Maesawa, C., Akasaka, T., and Masuda, T. Aberrant expression of the maspin gene associated with epigenetic modification in melanoma cells. J Invest Dermatol, 122: 805-811, 2004.
80. Xia, W., Lau, Y.K., Hu, M.C., Li, L., Johnston, D.A., Sheng, S., El-Naggar, A., and Hung, M.C. High tumoral maspin expression is associated with improved survival of patients with oral squamous cell carcinoma. Oncogene, 19: 2398-2403, 2000.
81. Yasumatsu, R., Nakashima, T., Hirakawa, N., Kumamoto, Y., Kuratomi, Y., Tomita, K., and Komiyama, S. Maspin expression in stage I and II oral tongue squamous cell carcinoma. Head Neck, 23: 962-966, 2001.
82. Navarro Rde, L., Martins, M.T., and de Araujo, V.C. Maspin expression in normal and neoplastic salivary gland. J Oral Pathol Med, 33: 435-440, 2004.
83. Sugimoto, S., Maass, N., Takimoto, Y., Sato, K., Minei, S., Zhang, M., Hoshikawa, Y., Junemann, K.P., Jonat, W., and Nagasaki, K. Expression and regulation of tumor suppressor gene maspin in human bladder cancer. Cancer Lett, 203: 209-215, 2004.
84. Friedrich, M.G., Toma, M.I., Petri, S., Cheng, J.C., Hammerer, P., Erbersdobler, A., and Huland, H. Expression of Maspin in non-muscle invasive bladder carcinoma: correlation with tumor angiogenesis and prognosis. Eur Urol, 45: 737-743, 2004.
85. Wentzensen, N., Wilz, B., Findeisen, P., Wagner, R., Dippold, W., von Knebel Doeberitz, M., and Gebert, J. Identification of differentially expressed genes in colorectal adenoma compared to normal tissue by suppression subtractive hybridization. Int J Oncol, 24: 987-994, 2004.
86. Song, S.Y., Lee, S.K., Kim, D.H., Son, H.J., Kim, H.J., Lim, Y.J., Lee, W.Y., Chun, H.K., and Rhee, J.C. Expression of maspin in colon cancers: its relationship with p53 expression and microvessel density. Dig Dis Sci, 47: 1831-1835, 2002.
87. Strathdee, G., Davies, B.R., Vass, J.K., Siddiqui, N., and Brown, R. Cell type-specific methylation of an intronic CpG island controls expression of the MCJ gene. Carcinogenesis, 25: 693-701, 2004.
88. Strathdee, G., Sim, A., and Brown, R. Control of gene expression by CpG island methylation in normal cells. Biochem Soc Trans, 32: 913-915, 2004.
89. Jones, P.A. and Taylor, S.M. Cellular differentiation, cytidine analogs and DNA methylation. Cell, 20: 85-93., 1980.
90. Taylor, S.M. and Jones, P.A. Multiple new phenotypes induced in 10T1/2 and 3T3 cells treated with 5- azacytidine. Cell, 17: 771-779., 1979.
91. Cameron, E.E., Bachman, K.E., Myohanen, S., Herman, J.G., and Baylin, S.B. Synergy of demethylation and histone deacetylase inhibition in the re-expression of genes silenced in cancer. Nat Genet, 21: 103-107, 1999.

Chapter 8

CELL ADHESION-MEDIATED RADIATION RESISTANCE: THE ROLE OF INTEGRINS AND INTEGRIN PROXIMAL PROTEIN

Nils Cordes
OcoRay-Radiation Research in Oncology, Medical Faculty Carl Gustav Carus, University of Technology, Dresden, Germany

Abstract: Existent or acquired resistance of tumor cells against genotoxic agents such as ionizing radiation or cytotoxic drugs is a widespread and clinically highly relevant phenomenon. Identifying cell-extracellular matrix interactions as critical, survival-improving factors within cellular resistance for normal and tumor cells has promoted intense research in this field. This chapter summarizes current and emerging data on how the molecular players such as integrins and intracellular protein kinases such as integrin-linked kinase and focal adhesion kinase coordinate signaling events for the cellular survival and growth response in DNA-damaged cells adherent to matrix proteins. Uncovering the molecular mechanisms may help to dissect central survival regulators in normal versus tumor tissue, which would provide the necessary knowledge for developing further innovative molecular-targeted anticancer strategies.

Key words: CAM-RR; CAM-DR; integrins; radiosensitivity; ECM; ILK; FAK

Abbreviations: ECM, extracellular matrix; ILK, integrin-linked kinase; AKT, protein kinase B/AKT; IR, ionizing radiation; FAK, focal adhesion kinase; MAPK, mitogen-activated protein kinase; PI3K, phosphatidylinositol-3-kinase; CAM-DR, cell adhesion-mediated drug resistance; CAM-RR, cell adhesion-mediated radioresistance.

1. INTRODUCTION

Cell-matrix interactions are in majority mediated by the integrin family of cell adhesion molecules. To date, 24 distinguishable transmembrane

A.E. Cress and R.B. Nagle (eds.), Cell Adhesion and Cytoskeletal Molecules in Metastasis, 141–162.

heterodimers consistent of one α and one β integrin subunit have been identified (1). Dependent on cell type and cellular context one out of 18 α and one out of 8 β subunits bind to form an integrin receptor (1). Besides the ability to bind proteins of the extracellular matrix (ECM) such as fibronectin, collagen or laminin, some integrins recognize members of the ADAM (A Disintegrin And Metalloproteinase) family or counter receptors on neighboring cells such as immunoglobulin-type receptors like ICAMs (intercellular cell adhesion molecule) or VCAMs (vascular cell adhesion molecule) (2).

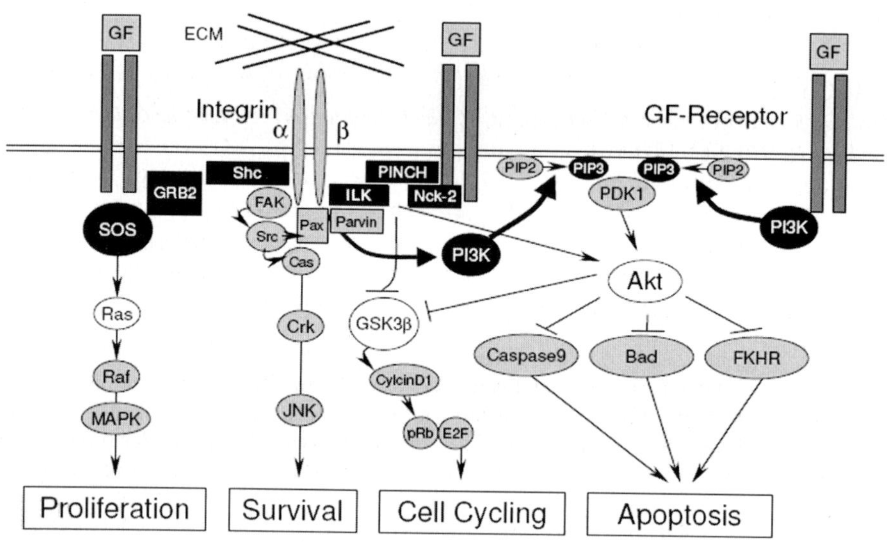

Figure 1. Some of the major pathways affected by integrin- and growth factor receptor-mediated signaling. In this schematic of the edge of a cell, the indicated molecules are located at the cell membrane for serving in signal transduction to downstream pathways. *In vivo*, this can be achieved by mutual and cooperate activation of regulatory cascades for cell survival, proliferation, cell cycling or apoptosis. It is illustrated non-comprehensively how critical protein kinases involved in the cellular response to genotoxic injury such as Akt, GSK3β, Src, MAPK and caspases are integrated into the intracellular network controlled by integrins and growth factor receptors. GF, growth factor.

In normal tissue, integrin-mediated cell-matrix interactions located at distinct membrane areas, termed focal adhesions, are indispensable for embryonic development and tissue integrity (3). Multiprotein complexes consisting of integrins, growth factor receptors, and adapter and signaling proteins assemble focal adhesions (4). Dissociation of the integrin-ECM interaction resulting in disassembly of focal adhesions and activation of matrix-degrading proteases enables cell detachment for migration and tissue remodeling. Further, integrin-mediated signaling cooperatively alters signaling induced by growth factors, cytokines or hormones for the regulation of downstream signaling pathways involved in cell survival, proliferation and differentiation (5-8) (Figure 1). Connecting protein kinases between kinase-lacking integrins and intracellular pathways are, for example, integrin-linked kinase (ILK) (9) and focal adhesion kinase (FAK) (10). Additional pathways and functions regulated by integrin-mediated adhesion are the phosphatidylinositol-3-kinase (PI3K)/Akt pathway, Ras/mitogen-activated protein kinase pathway, activation of transcription factors like NFκB, inositol lipid metabolism, Na^+/H^+ antiporter as well as matrix metalloproteinase activity (11).

Integrins and integrin-mediated signal transduction are also highly relevant in oncogenic transformation and tumor growth as highlighted through studies on cytoskeletal disorganization, attenuated cell adhesion, anchorage-independent cell survival and growth and alteration of integrin-mediated signaling (2, 12-15). Dependent on the tumor and integrin subtype, the changes in expression either promote or suppress the transformed phenotype. A promoting effect has been observed for integrin α6β4 in a subset of transformed breast epithelial cells (16,) as well as in carcinomas of the colon, skin and the head and neck region (13). The reduction of integrin α6β4 was associated with the conversion of normal prostate glands to carcinoma in-situ and invasive tumors in patients with prostate cancer (16 - 18). A suppressive effect of integrin expression on oncogenic transformation was discovered for the fibronectin receptor α5β1 (19). Whereas transformation of rodent fibroblasts by Src or Ras causes disappearance of α5β1 integrin from the cell surface and decline of fibronectin synthesis, overexpression of α5β1 integrin overrides the transformed phenotype and impairs tumor formation in immunodeficient mice. One potential mediator of this action seems to be the frequently mutated tumor suppressor protein $p16^{INK4a}$, which induces α5 integrin gene transcription (20). In general, changes in integrin expression associated with oncogenic transformation are a spatial disarrangement in the integrin cell surface pattern that influences ligand binding affinity, elevate glycosylation and phosphorylation of integrins (21, 22).

The aforementioned facts clearly demonstrate that integrin-mediated cell-matrix interactions are strong regulators of tumor cell behavior. On this basis, several studies have elucidated how these interactions modulate cellular chemo- and radiation sensitivity (23-29). The *in vitro* and *in vivo* observations clearly emphasize the clinical relevance of cell adhesion-mediated radiation (CAM-RR) and drug (CAM-DR) resistance inevitably linked to aggravated tumor control or treatment failure. In the following, I illustrate recent emerging findings concerning integrin-mediated alteration of survival and apoptosis particularly in tumor cells following genotoxic injury.

1.1 The Pro-Survival Effects of Cell-Matrix Interactions in Cells Stressed by Cytotoxic Drugs or Ionizing Radiation

Intriguingly, most clinically used chemotherapeutic agents tested in *in vitro* studies are less cytotoxic in matrix adhered cells. Early work was performed in small cell lung cancer (SCLC) cells on matrigel (solubilized basement membrane preparation extracted from Engelbreth-Holm-Swarm mouse sarcoma) or laminin showing reduced cytotoxicity of etoposide, cisplatin and doxorubicin (30). In the same tumor entity, Sethi et al. (26) and Kraus et al. (31) demonstrated impaired caspase-3 or Akt induction, respectively, by β1-integrin-mediated adhesion to fibronectin or laminin after etoposide, cyclophosphamide or doxorubicin treatment. Not unique to SCLC, resistance-promoting effects by integrin-mediated adhesion to ECM were also found in tumors of colon, pancreas (29), ovary (32), prostate (33), breast (34), liver (35) and brain (36). Most interestingly, leukemia cells show similar reduction of drug- and radiation-induced apoptosis upon adhesion to matrix proteins (37, 38).

Efforts to uncover the underlying mechanisms and central molecular players yielded a large variety of potential candidates starting with integrins, integrin signaling mediators such as ILK or FAK, p53, p27, $p16^{INK4a}$, Akt or Bcl-2 (24, 38-42). However, due to the large number of integrin receptors, complex intracellular signaling networks and mutual cooperation between integrin- and growth factor receptor-mediated signal transduction pathways, the identification of these players strongly emphasizes integrin-mediated modification of probably all pathways critically involved in the cellular response to genotoxic injury.

An open question deals with tumor-stroma interactions and how this interrelationship impacts on ECM deposition, integrin expression and signaling. Fast growing tumor tissue indicates a high turnover rate in active remodeling of the ECM within and adjacent to the tumor (43, 44). Herein, massive growth factor release and neovascularization are steps to be considered in the development of tumor cell drug resistance. ECM bound growth factors could be essential nutrients for migrating tumor cells on their way to blood vessels or drug-free/reduced tumor areas where inside-out and outside-in signaling via integrins promotes genomic- or proteomic-based drug and radiation protection.

In the following, the involvement of integrins, ILK and FAK are expounded in detail as critical modulators of the cellular response to genotoxic injury and as potential candidates in molecular-targeted therapeutic strategies.

2. THE ROLE OF INTEGRINS FOR THE CELLULAR RESPONSE TO GENOTOXIC INJURY

Certain integrins seem to communicate increased drug resistance in a great variety of malignancies. α5β1 integrin, for example, seems to be a major antagonist of cell death induced by doxorubicin or melphalan in multiple myeloma (45), by paclitaxel in breast cancer or small cell and non small cell lung cancer (NSCLC) (46,47) or by cisplatin or mitomycin C in NSCLC (47). Studies accomplished in murine GD25 fibroblasts that express wild-type β1A integrins or mutant β1B integrins clearly reveal an essential regulatory function of the β1A integrin variant in the cellular radiation response (48,49). Upon binding to fibronectin, laminin or collagen-III, β1A but not β1B integrins control pro-survival signaling cascades, which results in similar radiation survival rates under growth factor presence as compared to growth factor depletion. Cell adhesion via functional β1A integrins rescued Akt-S473 and -T308, p130Cas-Y410 and paxillin-Y118/-Y31 phosphorylation and blocked JNK activation, thus, providing a strong molecular basis for β1 integrin-dependent improvement of cell survival after genotoxic injury. Confirmatory studies were performed in human A-172 glioma cells following siRNA-mediated silencing of β1 integrin expression.

Further regulatory pathways influenced by β1 integrins were uncovered that exert cellular resistance to genotoxic agents (24, 29, 48, 50). For example, β1 integrin-mediated cytoprotection against pharmacological DNA-damaging agents like bleomycin, etoposide or fludarabine has been associated with reduction of proapoptotic proteins Bim and Bax (37, 40, 51) in parallel with induction of antiapoptotic Bcl-2-like proteins or Bcl-2/Bax ratio (39).

With concern to cell cycle distribution, which critically affects the survival of cell cultures treated with genotoxic agents *in vitro*, the exact impact of the cell cycle distribution for drug and radiation survival is unclear *in vivo* (52-54). *In vitro* studies using normal and tumor cell lines clearly showed that cells in the G1 cell cycle phase are significantly less chemo- and radiosensitive than proliferating cells in S or G2.

Under drug treatment, S-phase cells increasingly incorporate the DNA analog or DNA intercalating substance. This results in the termination of DNA replication or DNA damage repair. Ionizing radiation faces a larger DNA molecule in S and G2/M phase cells for the indirect infliction of various DNA lesions (55). The main lesions are single or double strand breaks, base damage or clustered lesions. After irradiation, cells are blocked in cell cycle phases G1 or G2. DNA damage recognition and repair enzymes such as Ataxia-telangiectasia-mutated gene (ATM) or checkpoint kinases, cyclins, cyclin-dependent kinases (CDK) and cyclin-dependent kinase inhibitors tightly regulate these processes (56).

Considering these aspects, growth of cells on ECM proteins prolongs the radiation-induced cell cycle arrest at the G1- and G2 checkpoints as compared to cells growing on non-specific substrata (57-60). In general, this delay at the different cell cycle checkpoints after genotoxic injury is believed to provide more time for DNA damage repair, which accomplishes genomic integrity of daughter cells prior to continuing cell cycle transition and mitogenesis (61-63). Investigations in A-549 human lung carcinoma cells and human fibroblasts exhibited an increase in the basal phosphorylation of the checkpoint kinases Chk1 and Chk2 (59). The DNA damage recognition and repair protein complex Ku70/Ku80 (64) and the poly(ADP-ribose) polymerase (PARP) (65) are strongly affected by integrin-ECM interactions, since Ku70/Ku80 might represent a new cell surface receptor for fibronectin and PARP regulates chromatin structure in an integrin activity-dependent manner. The latter interrelation was particularly examined in bleomycin-treated PARP knockout mouse lung epithelial cells. Activation of these DNA repair pathways by integrin-mediated adhesion to matrix *per se* is likely to accelerate DNA damage removal and/or to optimize the efficacy of DNA damage repair after irradiation for providing genomic integrity and thus cell survival.

Searching for specific integrins in CAM-RR or -DR, Kremer et al. (66) found a dependence of radiation-induced G2 cell cycle arrest in human prostate epithelial but not prostate epithelial cancer cells on $\alpha6\beta4$ integrin and its ligand laminin 5. With respect to $\beta1$ integrin, we recently reported significant basal accumulation of mutant $\beta1B$ integrin expressing GD25$\beta1B$ and human $\beta1$ integrin knockdown A-172 glioma cells but not wild-type $\beta1A$ integrin expressing GD25$\beta1A$ cells in the G1-phase under serum depletion (49). However, this increased amount of G1 cells could not be correlated with an improvement in radiation survival of GD25$\beta1B$ cells but rather with elevated cell killing.

In addition to communicating survival advantage and cell cycle modifying effects in cells seeded onto ECM proteins prior to drug or radiation treatment, integrins themselves are affected by ionizing radiation.

Following radiation exposure, the expression of several integrin subunits including β1-, β3, α5, αv- is upregulated in human skin and lung fibroblasts (29), endothelial cells and keratinocytes (67) as well as in tumor cells of the lung (27), brain (68), colon, hematopoetic cells (69), pancreas (70) and melanomas (29). The underlying molecular mechanisms and consequences of these alterations are currently unclear. However, one elegant therapeutic approach used enhancement of αvβ3 integrin expression on sublethally irradiated endothelial cells. Herewith, drugs or immunoradioisotopes were directly delivered into the irradiated and proliferating endothelium of GL261 gliomas and B16F0 melanoma implanted into C57BL6 mice (71). This might be a reasonable strategy for tumor-specific integrin targeting in selected tumor entities.

Brown et al. (72) showed that radiation-dependent increase in αv- and β1-integrin in HUVEC is strictly coupled to the presence of U87 glioma cells. This observation adds a new facet to the tumor-promoting impact of tumor stroma, tumor-stroma crosstalk and the role normal tissue is likely to play in the reaction of cancer cells to genotoxic compounds.

Subsequent to fractionated irradiation of prostate carcinoma cells with a total dose of 25 Gy applied within 3 weeks, Simon et al. (70) observed a reduction in β1-integrin expression and concomitant decrease in cell proliferation. Similarly, exposing cells to commonly administered genotoxic drugs such as cisplatin, 5'-fluorouracil or cyclophosphamide generally results in decreased integrin expression as a consequence of apoptosis induction. Nevertheless, there is a lack of detailed studies elucidating long-term, time-dependent changes in integrin expression under genotoxic agents. Eventually, these clinical and translation research-related radiation schedules shed light on possible therapeutic intervention using anti-integrin and/or adhesion-blocking agents.

Besides regulating survival and proliferation, the radiation-induced integrin cell surface expression improves cell adhesion and might also affect migration. Studies in glioma cells elucidating these features with regard to possible therapeutic consequences showed controversial results. A 3.5-Gy irradiation of U87-MG, LN-18 and LN-229 glioma cells enhanced cell migration and invasion into fetal rat brain (73). Irradiating the same cell lines (LN-18, LN-229) and others (A-172, U-138MG glioma cells) with 6 Gy revealed, however, a significant increase in cell adhesion and inhibition of cell invasion into matrigel, which was regulated by β1- and β3-integrins (68). Under both conditions, radiation-dependent induction of MMP-2 and -9 expression and activity was detectable but exerted opposing effects. Taken into account the higher rate of cell killing after 6 Gy versus 3.5 Gy, one could imagine that 3.5 Gy activate MMPs to a lesser extent than 6 Gy. Thus,

MMP-dependent matrix degradation is rather moderate following the lower radiation dose and still provides attachment points for integrins during migration. In contrast, matrix proteolysis by MMPs after higher doses of ionizing radiation is largely eradicating potent integrin ligands for cell migration. In combination with increased integrin cell surface presentation, local cell anchorage is, at least transiently, enforced.

3. THE ROLE OF INTEGRIN-MEDIATED SIGNALING MOLECULES FOR THE CELLULAR REACTION TO GENOTOXIC INJURY

Recruitment of cytoplasmic protein kinases and adapter proteins is necessary for integrin signal transduction to regulate cell survival, proliferation, differentiation as well as damage repair following genotoxic injury. FAK and ILK, as essential integrin signaling mediators, are the most intensively examined protein kinases in cells after genotoxic stress.

3.1 Focal Adhesion Kinase (FAK)

Combined immunohistochemical and molecular analysis of tumor specimens has demonstrated a pivotal role of the non-receptor bound FAK in a variety of human neoplasias. In lung cancer (74), hepatocellular carcinoma (75), squamous cell carcinoma (76), breast cancer (77), thyroid cancer (78), ovarian cancer (79) and astrocytoma (80), (FAK) expression and phosphorylation were elevated indicating that FAK might be a novel therapeutic target, prognostic marker and potential indicator for oncogenic transformation.

Kasahara et al. (41) was the first to examine the function of FAK in cellular coping mechanisms upon genotoxic injury. They showed that FAK overexpression prevents DNA fragmentation and caspase-3 and -8 activation, which consequently impaired radiation-induced apoptosis in human HL-60 leukemia cells. In parallel, FAK induced antiapoptotic PI3K/Akt signaling and the expression of the inhibitor-of-apoptosis proteins cIAP-2 and XIAP. In addition to radiation resistance, upregulated FAK protected HL-60 cells against hydrogen peroxide-, etoposide- or TRAIL-induced apoptosis (81).

Experiments using adherent growing A-549 lung carcinoma cells revealed that particularly the FAK-Y397 autophosphorylation site and FAK-Y925 facilitating complex formation with Grb2/SOS were increasingly phosphorylated after irradiation (82). In contrast, FAK-Y576, which is substantial for maximum kinase activity, was not activated after irradiation. Assuming that elevated phosphorylation of protein kinases determines increased signaling activity, FAK and its interacting partners p130Cas and paxillin play a crucial role in the cellular radiation response. One possible explanation for the enhanced phosphorylation of these proteins is the fact that the ionizing radiation produces a large amount of reactive oxygen species (ROS) (83). Zent et al. (84) showed that, in general, ROS initiate increased phosphorylation of various focal adhesion proteins including FAK.

Treatment of cells with cytotoxic drugs, however, exerts a different picture with regard to cell death and phosphorylation of focal adhesion proteins. Drug-treated cells die via different forms of programmed cell death (85), which all eventually initiate cell detachment from the substratum. During this process, integrins and other cell adhesion molecules are shed from the cell membrane and focal adhesions together with the associated multiprotein membrane complexes are disassembled (86). Studies performed in human hepatoma Hep3B cells treated with all-trans-retinoic acid (87) or bone marrow and dermal derived endothelial cells exposed to etoposide (88) underscore this differential cell response pattern upon drug exposure as compared with irradiation. Despite the current lack of definite mechanistic conclusions, FAK and its related proteins are modulated after irradiation and elevated FAK levels confer radioprotective effects, especially via antiapoptotic proteins as characterized through proteome analysis (89). In conjunction with FAK´s role in tumor growth and metastatic spread, the FAK/p130Cas/paxillin signaling complex might turn out as potential target for small molecule inhibitors in anticancer therapy.

3.1.1 Integrin-linked kinase (ILK)

ILK, an important β1-integrin signaling mediator, shows increased expression in prostate cancer (90), NSCLC (91), colon cancer (92), gastric cancer (93), ovarian cancer (94) and melanoma (95). These findings, in similarity to FAK, have led to regarding ILK as a novel therapeutic target and marker in prognosis and carcinogenesis.

ILK serves in survival/apoptosis and growth regulation via Akt/caspase-3 and -8 and GSK3β in IEC-18 rat intestinal cell, 293 human embryonic kidney cells and SCP2 mouse mammary epithelial cells (96-98). Under cellular stress caused by cytotoxic drugs or ionizing radiation, ILK transduces opposing effects as compared to FAK. Likewise in A-549 lung carcinoma and FaDu squamous cell carcinoma cells, elevated constitutive kinase-active ILK caused alteration of PI3K/Akt, GSK3β and MAPK signaling (47; Eke and Cordes, unpublished observations, 2005). Augmented ILK expression enforced cytoplasmic rather then membrane localization of ILK itself and its binding partners α-parvin and PINCH-1 (particularly interesting new cysteine-histidine rich protein 1) (99-100). Absence of ILK/α-parvin/PINCH-1 complex membrane localization initiated a decline in the number of focal adhesions and a fibroblastoid morphology characterized by enhanced formation of undirected filopodia. Moreover, integrin clustering and cell adhesion were perturbed in constitutive kinase-active ILK transfectants. Further evidence that ILK manifests elevated sensitivity to external cytotoxic stimuli was found in FAK deficient HL-60 cells (Hess, Estrugo, Fischer, Cordes, unpublished observations, 2004). Adhesion of this leukemia cell line to fibronectin promoted radiation-induced apoptosis via interaction of ILK with caspase-8.

ILK does not *per se* mediate increased cell killing after gentotoxic injury as recently demonstrated by Duxbury et al. (101). The authors found that overexpressed ILK protects pancreatic adenocarcinoma cells from undergoing apoptosis induced by the clinically administered anticancer drug and nucleoside analogue gemcitabine. ILK knockdown, however, resulted in an Akt- and caspase-3-dependent initiation of apoptosis. Future studies already underway will shed light on these inconsistent observations.

Another approach to elucidate the function of ILK in cell death regulation employed antisense transfection or different small molecule inhibitors against ILK (101-104). Anticancer effects of silenced or inhibited ILK were mediated by decreased Akt-S473 phosphorylation in glioblastoma cells *in vitro*. *In vivo*, ILK inhibition also abrogated PI3K/Akt phosphorylation, which subsequently modified the mammalian target of rapamycin (mTOR), signal transducers and activators of transcription 3 (STAT3) and forkhead transcription factors in tumor growth inhibition experiments using an orthotopic primary xenograft model of pancreatic cancer (104).

Overall, ILK presents as another focal adhesion associated protein kinase to be favorably targeted by molecular therapeutics in a variety of human malignancies. This view is underscored by the fact that the expression and localization of the ILK binding partners PINCH-1, α-parvin and Nck-2 greatly depend on the proper function of ILK (100). Therapeutically modifying ILK is, therefore, likely to result in the effective disruption of integrin-mediated as well as growth factor receptor-mediated pro-survival signaling.

4. THERAPEUTIC IMPACT OF TARGETED APPROACHES AGAINST MOLECULES INVOLVED IN CELL-MATRIX INTERACTIONS

Reviewing the role of integrins and integrin-associated structural and signaling molecules in the cellular survival and growth responses upon genotoxic injury raises the question whether the modification or targeting of these proteins could potentially improve anticancer treatment strategies.

In general, small molecule inhibitors, gene therapy, antibodies or short peptidomimetics are imaginable ways to target the major players constituting focal adhesions (105-109).

Detailed knowledge about integrin expression and function has been collected in different model systems *in vitro* and *in vivo*. The examination of integrin expression patterns in normal and tumor tissue has provided useful insight into integrin distribution in different healthy tissues as compared to tumor stroma and the tumor itself. To optimize multimodal therapeutic approaches using the new molecular therapeutics outlined above, intense molecular and imaging studies are advised to clarify the exact target(s) of a specific signal transduction modulator. Fundamentally, the presence of the targeted molecule in the tumor cell or in the tumor-associated stroma seems to be demanded but not sufficient for the anticancer efficacy of such agents.

Table 1 gives a short overview about currently undertaken clinical trials administering approved or non-approved anti-integrin antibodies or short peptidomimetics. The upcoming years will reveal the potential and therapeutic index of such exciting novel molecular compounds alone, in co-administration with conventional anticancer drugs, radiotherapy or agents directed against other cell surface receptors and intracellular molecules.

5. CONCLUSIONS

An aggravating factor to be considered in cytotoxicity studies is that cell-matrix interactions as well as focal adhesion formation are different under two-dimensional versus three-dimensional cell culture conditions. These circumstances have to be deeply elucidated in the future to pinpoint significant differences in the regulation of coping mechanisms for genotoxic injury in these two cell culture models. Although *in vivo* studies will keep

Table 1. Anti-integrin compounds in cancer and other diseases in current clinical trials or on the market (M).

Agent	Commercial Name	Company	Type of Agent	Target	Disease	Trial status	Reference
AN100226m Natalizumab	Antegren, Tysabri	Elan Corporation	mAb, humanized	CD49d (VLA-4) integrin α4β1	Acute and chronic inflammatory diseases (e.g. rheumatoid arthritis)	Phase III	www.elan.com
AN100226m Natalizumab	Antegren, Tysabri	AERES Biomedical	mAb, humanized	CD49d (VLA-4) integrin α4β1	Multiple sclerosis	Phase III, M	Leger 1997, Miller 2003, Rice 2005
AN100226m Natalizumab	Antegren, Tysabri	Athena Neurosciences, Tysabri, Biogen Idec, Elan	mAb, humanized	CD49d (VLA-4) integrin α4β1	Colitis, Crohn´s disease	Phase II	www.elan.com
LDP-02, MLN-02		Genentech, Millenium	mAb, humanized	integrin α4β7 (LPAM-1)	inflammatory bowel disease	Phase II	Cordes 2005
BIO-1211		Biogen, Merck & Co	Peptide	Integrin α4β1 (VLA-4)	allergy, asthma	Phase II	Cordes 2005
RT-14035, SB683698		Tanabe Seiyaku, GlaxoSmithKline	Non-peptide	Integrin α4β1 (VLA-4), Integrin α4β7 (LPAM-1)	asthma, inflammatory bowel disease, multiple sclerosis	Phase II	Cordes 2005
HU23F2G, 23F2G	LeukArrest	Icos	mAb, chimeric human-mouse (IgG4)	CD11, integrin β2, integrin αLβ2 (LFA-1)	ischaemic stroke	Phase III	Cordes 2005
	Erlizumab	Genentech, Roche	mAb, human-mouse light chain dimer	human CD18, integrin αLβ2 (LFA-1)	ischaemic stroke, acute myocardial infarction	Phase II	Baran 2001
	Abciximab	Centocor	mAb	Integrin αvβ3	Angina pectoris	M	Topol 1994
Tirofiban	Aggrastat		synthetic compound, non-peptide, mimic of RGD	Integrin α2β3	Acute coronary syndromes	M	Tscheng 1996, Alexander 1998, Weintraub 1999
EMD121974	Cilengitide	Merck KGaA	small molecule blocker	Integrin αXβ3	Kaposi´s sarcoma		Eskens 2000
EMD121974	Cilengitide	Merck KGaA	small molecule blocker	Integrin αXβ3	renal cell carcinoma, colon cancer	Phase I	Eskens 2000
EMD121974	Cilengitide	Merck KGaA	small molecule blocker	Integrin αXβ3	recurrent or progressive malignant gliomas	Phase I	www.clinicaltrials.gov
EMD121974	Cilengitide	Merck KGaA	small molecule blocker	Integrin αXβ3	Newly diagnosed glioblastoma multiforme	Phase I/II	www.clinicaltrials.gov
EMD121974	Cilengitide	Merck KGaA	small molecule blocker	Integrin αXβ3	Malignant melanoma	Phase II	www.clinicaltrials.gov

Agent	Commercial Name	Company	Type of Agent	Target	Disease	Trial status	Reference
eptifibatide	Integrilin	Millenium Pharmaceuticals	Cyclic heptapeptide containing KGD sequence	Integrin α2bβ3	Acute coronary syndrome	M	www.mlnm.com
EMD 121974	Cilengitide	EMD Pharmaceuticals, Merck KGaA	mAb	Integrin αvβ3 and αvβ5	Glioblastoma multiforme	Phase II	www.clinicaltrials.gov
EMD 121974	Cilengitide	EMD Pharmaceuticals, Merck KGaA	mAb	Integrin αvβ3 and αvβ5	Advanced solid tumors or lymphomas	Phase I	www.clinicaltrials.gov
EMD 121974	Cilengitide	EMD Pharmaceuticals, Merck KGaA	mAb	Integrin αvβ3 and αvβ5	Acute myeloid leukaemia (AML)	Phase II	www.clinicaltrials.gov
	Thalidomide		small molecule agent	Integrin αv and β3 promoter	malignant gliomas	Phase II	www.clinicaltrials.gov
MLN01 (LDP-01)		Millenium Pharmaceuticals	mAb	Integrin α2	Cardiovascular diseases, thrombosis, stroke	Phase I/II	www.mlnm.com
MLN02		Millenium Pharmaceuticals	mAb, humanized	Integrin α4β7	Crohn´s disease	Phase II	www.mlnm.com
MLN02		Millenium Pharmaceuticals	mAb, humanized	Integrin α4β7	Ulcerative colitis	Phase II	www.mlnm.com
M200	Volociximab	Protein Design Labs	mAb	Integrin α5β1	renal cell carcinoma metastases	Phase II	www.clinicaltrials.gov
M200	Volociximab	Protein Design Labs	mAb	Integrin α5β1	Melanoma metastases (combination with DTIC)	Phase II	http://utm-ext01a.mdacc.tmc.edu, www.clinicaltrials.gov
MEDI-525		MedImmune Inc.	mAb	Integrin αvβ3	refractory advanced solid tumors, Leukemia, Lymphoma, small intestine cancer	Phase I	www.clinicaltrials.gov
MEDI-522	Vitaxin	MedImmune Inc.	mAb	Integrin αvβ3	metastatic malignant melanoma	Phase II	www.clinicaltrials.gov
MEDI-522	Vitaxin	MedImmune Inc.	mAb	Integrin αvβ3	rheumatoid arthritis	Phase II	www.clinicaltrials.gov
MEDI-522	Vitaxin	MedImmune Inc.	mAb	Integrin αvβ3	metastatic androgen-independent prostate cancer, combination therapy	Phase II	www.clinicaltrials.gov
MEDI-522	Vitaxin	MedImmune Inc.	mAb	Integrin αvβ3	malignant melanoma	Phase I	www.clinicaltrials.gov
MEDI-522	Vitaxin	MedImmune Inc.	mAb	Integrin αvβ3	plaque psoriasis	Phase II	www.clinicaltrials.gov
Ro 27-2441		Hoffmann-la Roche		dual integrin antagonist	Asthma	Phase II	www.clinicaltrials.gov
Ro 27-2771		Hoffmann-la Roche		dual integrin antagonist	Asthma	Phase II	www.clinicaltrials.gov

their eligibility as final preclinical experiment, it can be hypothesized that optimized cell culture conditions can substantially foster anticancer drug identification and development.

Concerning existent or acquired cellular drug and radiation resistance, integrin-mediated cell-ECM interactions are very likely to play an essential role in combination with survival-advantaging genetic mutations in e.g. epidermal growth factor receptor gene (110), multidrug resistance gene 1

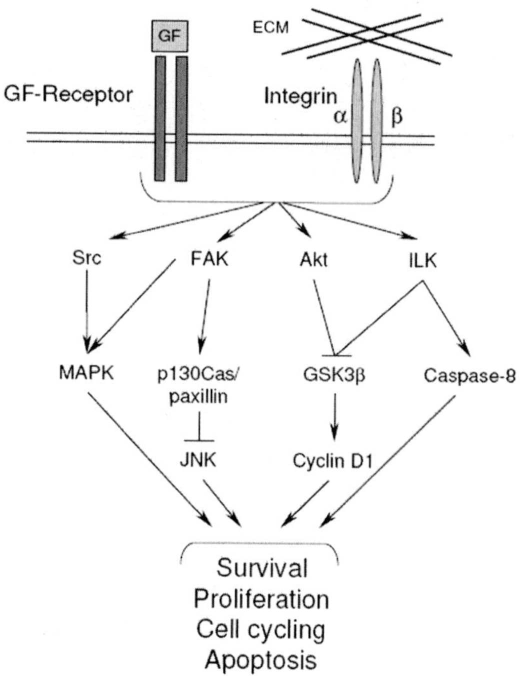

Figure 2. Schematic diagram depicting specific focal adhesion proteins in the cellular genotoxic stress response examined in more detail during the last years. Although integrin and growth factor receptor interactions coordinately control e.g., cell survival and growth, the exact molecular processes taken place after DNA damage are largely unclear to date. However, integrin-mediated cell adhesion to extracellular matrix proteins channels through the indicated structural and signaling molecules for attenuating the cellular chemo- and radiation sensitivity of two-dimensional human and murine cell cultures.

(MDR1; associated with p-glycoprotein) (111) or BCR-Abl-kinase (112) (Figure 2). Integrin receptors and their downstream signaling mediators anticipate challenging and effective targets for innovative therapeutic strategies directed against the primary tumor as well as its metastases. Future investigations on tumor-specific integrin-mediated signaling and their crosstalk with growth factor receptor-mediated signaling may also substantially contribute to the identification of new molecular targets and the development of interacting substances for adjuvant chemo- and radiotherapy strategies.

ACKNOWLEDGEMENTS

Part of the work in the author's laboratory was funded by the Federal Ministry of Education, Science, Research and Technology (BMBF-03ZIK041). The author thanks Dr. Stephanie Hehlgans, Dr. Michael Haase and Mr. Steffen Kausch for critical reading of the manuscript and for the overview on clinical trials administering anti-integrin agents. I am further grateful to Ms. Iris Eke and Mr. Veit Sandfort for the schematic drawings.

REFERENCES

1. Hynes, R.O., 2002, Integrins: Bidirectional, allosteric signaling machines, Cell 110:673-687.
2. Danen, E.H., 2005, Integrins: regulators of tissue function and cancer progression, Curr. Pharm. Des. 11:881-891.
3. Wozniak, M.A., Modzelewska, K., Kwong, L., and Keely, P.J., 2004, Focal adhesion regulation of cell behavior, Biochim. Biophys. Acta 1692:103-119.
4. Hauck, C.R., Hsia, D.A., and Schlaepfer, D.D., 2002, The focal adhesion kinase--a regulator of cell migration and invasion, IUBMB Life 53:115-119.
5. Watt, F.M., 2002, Role of integrins in regulating epidermal adhesion, growth and differentiation, EMBO J. 21:19-26.
6. Brakebusch, C., and Fässler, R., 2003, The integrin-actin connection, an eternal love affair, EMBO J. 22:2324-2333.
7. Comoglio, P.M., Boccaccio, C., and Trusolino, L., 2003, Interactions between growth factor receptors and adhesion molecules: breaking the rules, Curr. Opin. Cell Biol. 15:565-571.

8. Giancotti, F.G., and Tarone, G., 2003, Positional control of cell fate through joint integrin/receptor protein kinase signaling, Annu. Rev. Cell Dev. Biol. 19:173-206.
9. Hannigan, G.E., Leung-Hagesteijn, C., Fitz-Gibbon, L., Coppolino, M.G., Radeva, G., Filmus, J., Bell, J.C., and Dedhar, S., 1996, Regulation of cell adhesion and anchorage-dependent growth by a new β1-integrin-linked protein kinase, Nature 379:91-96.
10. Schaller, M.D., 2001, Biochemical signals and biological responses elicited by the focal adhesion kinase, Biochem. Biophys. Acta 1540:1-21.
11. Schwartz, M.A., 2001, Integrin signaling revisited, Trends Cell Biol. 12:466-470.
12. Ruoslahti, E., 1997, Integrins as signaling molecules and targets for tumor therapy, Kidney Int. 51:1413-1417.
13. Mizejewski, G.J., 1999, Role of integrins in cancer: survey of expression patterns, Proc. Soc. Exp. Biol. Med. 222:124-138.
14. Hanahan, D., and Weinberg, R.A., 2000, The hallmarks of cancer, Cell 100, 57-70.
15. Jin, H., and Varner, J., 2004, Integrins: roles in cancer development and as treatment targets, Brit. J. Cancer 90:561-565.
16. Davis, T.L., Cress, A.E., Dalkin, B.L., and Nagle, R.B., 2001, Unique expression pattern of the alpha6beta4 integrin and laminin-5 in human prostate carcinoma, Prostate 46:240-248.
17. Witkowski, C.M., Bowden, G.T., Nagle, R.B., and Cress, A.E., 2000, Altered surface expression and increased turnover of the alpha6beta4 integrin in an undifferentiated carcinoma, Carcinogenesis 21:325-330.
18. Cress, A.E., Rabinovitz, I., Zhu, W., and Nagle, R.B., 1995, The alpha 6 beta 1 and alpha 6 beta 4 integrins in human prostate cancer progression, Cancer Metastasis Rev. 14:219-228.
19. Chen, F.A., Repasky, E.A., and Bankert, R.B., 1991, Human lung tumor-associated antigen identified as an extracellular matrix adhesion molecule, J. Exp. Med. 173:1111-1119.
20. Plath, T., Detjen, K., Welzel, M., von Marschall, Z., Murphy, D., Schirner, M., Wiedenmann, B., and Rosewicz, S., 2000, A novel function for the tumor suppressor p16(INK4a): induction of anoikis via upregulation of the alpha(5)beta(1) fibronectin receptor, J. Cell Biol. 150:1467-1478.
21. Kashiwagi, H., Tomiyama, Y., Tadokoro, S., Honda, S., Shiraga, M., Mizutani, H., Handa, M., Kurata, Y., Matsuzawa, Y., and Shattil, S.J., 1999, A mutation in the extracellular cysteine-rich repeat region of the beta3 subunit activates integrins alphaIIbbeta3 and alphaVbeta3, Blood 93:2559-2568.
22. Guo, H.B., Lee, I., Bryan, B.T., and Pierce, M., 2005, Deletion of mouse embryo fibroblast N-acetylglucosaminyltransferase V stimulates alpha5beta1 integrin expression mediated by the protein kinase C signaling pathway, J. Biol. Chem. 280:8332-8342.
23. Fuks, Z., Vlodavsky, I., Andreeff, M., McLoughlin, M., and Haimovitz-Friedman, A., 1992, Effects of extracellular matrix on the response of endothelial cells to radiation in vitro, Eur. J. Cancer 28A:725-731.
24. Damiano, J.S., Cress, A.E., Hazlehurst, L.A., Shtil, A.A., and Dalton, W.S., 1999, Cell adhesion mediated drug resistance (CAM-DR): role of integrins and resistance to apoptosis in human myeloma cell lines, Blood 93:1658-1667.
25. Rose, R.W., Grant, D.S., O'Hara, M.D., and Williamson, S.K., 1999, The role of laminin-1 in the modulation of radiation damage in endothelial cells and differentiation, Radiat. Res. 152:14-28.

26. Sethi, T., Rintoul, R.C., Moore, S.M., MacKinnon, A.C., Salter, D., Choo, C., Chilvers, E.R., Dransfield, I., Donnelly, S.C., Strieter, R., and Haslett, C., 1999, Extracellular matrix proteins protect small cell lung cancer cells against apoptosis: a mechanism for small cell lung cancer growth and drug resistance in vivo, Nature Med 5:662-668.
27. Cordes, N., Blaese, M.A., Meineke, V., and van Beuningen, D., 2002, Ionizing radiation induces up-regulation of functional β1-integrin in lung tumour cell lines in vitro, Int. J. Radiat. Biol. 78:347-357.
28. Lewis, J.M., Truong, T.N., and Schwartz, M.A., 2002, Integrins regulate the apoptotic response to DNA damage through modulation of p53, Proc. Natl. Acad. Sci. USA 99:3627-3632.
29. Cordes, N., and Meineke, V., 2003, Cell adhesion-mediated radioresistance (CAM-RR): Extracellular matrix-dependent improvement of cell survival in human tumor and normal cells in vitro, Strahlenther. Onkol. 179:337-344.
30. Fridman, R., Giaccone, G., Kanemoto, T., Martin, G.R., Gazdar, A.F., and Mulshine, J.L., 1990. Reconstituted basement membrane (matrigel) and laminin can enhance the tumorigenicity and the drug resistance of small cell lung cancer cell lines, Proc. Natl. Acad. Sci. USA 87:6698-6702.
31. Kraus, A.C., Ferber, I., Bachmann, S.O., Specht, H., Wimmel, A., Gross, M.W., Schlegel, J., Suske, G., and Schuermann, M., 2002, In vitro chemo- and radio-resistance in small cell lung cancer correlates with cell adhesion and constitutive activation of AKT and MAP kinase pathways, Oncogene 21:8683-8695.
32. Maubant, S., Cruet-Hennequart, S., Poulain, L., Carreiras, F., Sichel, F., Luis, J., Staedel, C., Gauduchon, P., 2002, Altered adhesion properties and alphav integrin expression in a cisplatin-resistant human ovarian carcinoma cell line, Int. J. Cancer 97:186-194.
33. Miyamoto, H., Murakami, T., Tsuchida, K., Sugino, H., Miyake, H., and Tashiro, S., 2004, Tumor-stroma interaction of human pancreatic cancer: acquired resistance to anticancer drugs and proliferation regulation is dependent on extracellular matrix proteins, Pancreas 28:38-44.
34. Menendez, J.A., Vellon, L., Mehmi, I., Teng, P.K., Griggs, D.W., and Lupu, R., 2005, A novel CYR61-triggered 'CYR61-alphavbeta3 integrin loop' regulates breast cancer cell survival and chemosensitivity through activation of ERK1/ERK2 MAPK signaling pathway, Oncogene 24:761-779.
35. Zhang, H., Ozaki, I., Mizuta, T., Matsuhashi, S., Yoshimura, T., Hisatomi, A., Tadano, J., Sakai, T., and Yamamoto, K., 2002, Beta 1-integrin protects hepatoma cells from chemotherapy induced apoptosis via a mitogen-activated protein kinase dependent pathway, Cancer 95:896-906.
36. Uhm, J.H., Dooley, N.P., Kyritsis, A.P., Rao, J.S., and Gladson, C.L., 1999, Vitronectin, a glioma-derived extracellular matrix protein, protects tumor cells from apoptotic death, Clin. Cancer Res. 5:1587-1594.
37. Damiano, J.S., Hazlehurst, L.A., and Dalton, W.S., 2001, Cell adhesion-mediated drug resistance (CAM-DR) protects the K562 chronic myelogenous leukemia cell line from apoptosis induced by BCR/ABL inhibition, cytotoxic drugs, and gamma-irradiation, Leukemia 15:1232-1239.
38. de la Fuente, M.T., Casanova, B., Cantero, E., Hernandez del Cerro, M., Garcia-Marco, J., Silva, A., and Garcia-Pardo, A., 2003, Involvement of p53 in alpha4beta1 integrin-mediated resistance of B-CLL cells to fludarabine, Biochem. Biophys. Res. Commun. 311:708-712.

39. de la Fuente, M.T., Casanova, B., Garcia-Gila, M., Silva, A., and Garcia-Pardo, A., 1999, Fibronectin interaction with alpha4beta1 integrin prevents apoptosis in B cell chronic lymphocytic leukemia: correlation with Bcl-2 and Bax, Leukemia 13:266-274.
40. Hazlehurst, L.A., Damiano, J.S., Buyuksal, I., Pledger, W.J., and Dalton, W.S., 2000, Adhesion to fibronectin via β1-integrins regulates p27kip1 levels and contributes to cell adhesion mediated drug resistance (CAM-DR), Oncogene 19:4319-4327.
41. Kasahara, T., Koguchi, E., Funakoshi, M., Aizu-Yokota, E., and Sonoda, Y., 2002, Antiapoptotic action of focal adhesion kinase (FAK) against ionizing radiation, Antioxid. Redox Signal. 4:491-499.
42. Cordes, N., 2004, Overexpression of hyperactive integrin-linked kinase leads to increased cellular radiosensitivity, Cancer Res. 64:5683-5692.
43. Werb, Z., Vu, T.H., Rinkenberger, J.L., and Coussens, L.M., 1999, Matrix-degrading proteases and angiogenesis during development and tumor formation, APMIS 107:11-18.
44. Rundhaug, J.E., 2005, Matrix metalloproteinases and angiogenesis, J. Cell. Mol. Med. 9:267-285.
45. Hazlehurst, L.A., Valkov, N., Wisner, L., Storey, J.A., Boulware, D., Sullivan, D.M., and Dalton, W.S., 2001, Reduction in drug-induced DNA double-strand breaks associated with beta1 integrin-mediated adhesion correlates with drug resistance in U937 cells, Blood 98:1897-1903.
46. Aoudjit, F., and Vuori, K., 2001, Integrin signaling inhibits paclitaxel-induced apoptosis in breast cancer cells, Oncogene 20:4995-5004.
47. Cordes, N., Beinke, C., Plasswilm, L., and van Beuningen, D., 2004, Irradiation and various cytotoxic drugs enhance tyrosine phosphorylation and β1-integrin clustering in human A549 lung cancer cells in a substratum-dependent manner in vitro, Strahlenther. Onkol. 180:157-164.
48. Seidler, J., Durzok, R., Brakebusch, C., and Cordes, N., 2005, Interactions of the integrin subunit β1A with protein kinase B/Akt, p130Cas and paxillin contribute to regulation of radiation survival, Radiother. Oncol. 76:129-134.
49. Cordes, N., Seidler, J., Durzok, R., Geinitz, H., and Brakebusch, C., 2006, β1-integrin-mediated signaling essentially contributes to cell survival after radiation-induced genotoxic injury, Oncogene, in press.
50. Cordes, N., and van Beuningen, D., 2003, Cell adhesion to the extracellular matrix protein fibronectin modulates radiation-dependent G2 phase arrest involving integrin-linked kinase (ILK) and glycogen synthase kinase-3β (GSK-3β) in vitro, Brit. J. Cancer 88:1470-1479.
51. van der Kuip, H., Goetz, A.W., Miething, C., Duyster, J., and Aulitzky, W.E., 2001, Adhesion to fibronectin selectively protects Bcr-Abl+ cells from DNA damage-induced apoptosis, Blood 98:1532-1541.
52. Tubiana, M., 1982, L.H. Gray Medal lecture: cell kinetics and radiation oncology, Int. J. Radiat. Oncol. Biol. Phys. 8:1471-1489.
53. Tsang, R.W., Juvet, S., Pintilie, M., Hill, R.P., Wong, C.S., Milosevic, M., Chapman, W., Levin, W., Manchul, L.A., and Fykes, A.W., 2003, Pretreatment proliferation parameters do not add predictive power to clinical factors in cervical cancer treated with definitive radiation therapy, Clin. Cancer Res. 9:4387-4395.
54. Kirkpatrick, J.P., and Marks, L.B., 2004, Modeling killing and repopulation kinetics of subclinical cancer: direct calculations from clinical data, Int. J. Radiat. Oncol. Biol. Phys. 58:641-654.

55. Jackson, S.P., 2002, Sensing and repairing DNA double-strand breaks, Carinogenesis 23:687-696.
56. Pawlik, T.M., and Keyomarsi, K., 2004, Role of cell cycle in mediating sensitivity to radiotherapy, Int. J. Radiat. Oncol. Biol. Phys. 59:928-942.
57. Gadbois, D.M., Bradbury, E.M., and Lehnert, B.E., 1997, Control of radiation-induced G1 arrest by cell-substratum interactions, Cancer Res. 57:1151-1156.
58. Dimitrijevic-Bussod, M., Balzaretti-Maggi, V.S., and Gadbois, D.M., 1999, Extracellular matrix and radiation G1 cell cycle arrest in human fibroblasts, Cancer Res. 59:4843-4847.
59. Cordes, N., and van Beuningen, D., 2004, Arrest of human lung fibroblasts in G2 phase after irradiation is regulated by converging phosphatidylinositol-3 kinase and beta1-integrin signaling in vitro, Int. J. Radiat. Oncol. Biol. Phys. 58:453-462.
60. Cordes, N., and Beinke, C., 2004, Fibronectin alters A549 human lung cancer cell survival after irradiation, Cancer Biol. Ther. 3:47-53.
61. Little, J.B., and Nagasawa, H., 1985, Effect of confluent holding on potentially lethal damage repair, cell cycle progression, and chromosomal aberrations in human normal and ataxia-telangiectasia fibroblasts, Radiat. Res. 101:81-93.
62. Lane, D.P., 1992, Cancer. p53, guardian of the genome, Nature 358:15-16.
63. O′Connor, P.M., 1997, Mammalian G_1 and G_2 phase checkpoints, Cancer Surv. 29:151-182.
64. Monferran, S., Muller, C., Mourey, L., Frit, P., and Salles, B., 2004, The membrane-associated form of the DNA repair protein Ku is involved in cell adhesion to fibronectin, J. Mol. Biol. 337:503-511.
65. Jones, C.B., McIntosh, J., Huang, H., Graytock, A., and Hoyt, D.G., 2001, Regulation of bleomycin-induced DNA breakage and chromatin structure in lung endothelial cells by integrins and poly(ADP-ribose) polymerase, Mol. Pharmacol. 59:69-75.
66. Kremer, C.L., Schmelz, M., and Cress, A.E., 2005, Integrin-dependent amplification of the G2 arrest induced by ionizing radiation, Prostate 2006 Jan 1;66(1):88-96.
67. Meineke, V., Müller, K., Ridi, R., Cordes, N., Kohn, F.M., Mayerhofer, A., Ring, J., and van Beuningen, D., 2004, Development and evaluation of a skin organ model for the analysis of radiation effects, Strahlenther. Onkol. 180:102-108.
68. Cordes, N., Hansmeier, B., Beinke, C., Meineke, V., and van Beuningen, D., 2003, Irradiation differentially affects substratum-dependent survival, adhesion, and invasion of glioblastoma cell lines, Brit. J. Cancer 89:2122-2132.
69. Dong, L., Sun, H., Liu, W., Tao, D., Zhang, Y., and Xu, H., 1999, Effect of ligustrazine on expression of adherent molecule CD49d and cyclin D2 in hematopoietic cells in acute radiation injured mice, J. Tongji Med. Univ. 19:99-101.
70. Simon, E.L., Goel, H.L., Teider, N., Wang, T., Languino, L.R., and Fitzgerald, T.J., 2005, High dose fractionated ionizing radiation inhibits prostate cancer cell adhesion and beta(1) integrin expression, Prostate 64:83-91.
71. Hallahan, D., Geng, L., Qu, S., Scarfone, C., Giorgio, T., Donnelly, E., Gao, X., and Clanton, J., 2003, Integrin-mediated targeting of drug delivery to irradiated tumor blood vessels, Cancer Cell 3(1):63-74.
72. Brown, C.K., Khodarev, N.N., Yu, J., Moo-Young, T., Labay, E., Darga, T.E., Posner, M.C., Weichselbaum, R.R., and Mauceri, H.J., 2004, Glioblastoma cells block radiation-induced programmed cell death of endothelial cells, FEBS Lett. 565:167-170.
73. Wild-Bode, C., Weller, M., Rimner, A., Dichgans, J., and Wick, W., 2001, Sublethal irradiation promotes migration and invasiveness of glioma cells: implications for radiotherapy of human glioblastoma, Cancer Res. 61:2744-2750.

74. Wang, X.Y., Liu, T., Zhu, C.Z., Li, Y., Sun, R., Sun, C.Y., and Wang, A.X., 2005, Expression of KAI1, MRP-1, and FAK proteins in lung cancer detected by high-density tissue microarray, Ai Zheng 24:1091-1095.
75. Itoh, S., Maeda, T., Shimada, M., Aishima, S., Shirabe, K., Tanaka, S., and Maehara, Y., 2004, Role of expression of focal adhesion kinase in progression of hepatocellular carcinoma, Clin. Cancer Res. 10:2812-2817.
76. Aronsohn, M.S., Brown, H.M., Hauptman, G., and Kornberg, L.J., 2003, Expression of focal adhesion kinase and phosphorylated focal adhesion kinase in squamous cell carcinoma of the larynx, Laryngoscope 113:1944-1948.
77. Watermann, D.O., Gabriel, B., Jager, M., Orlowska-Volk, M., Hasenburg, A., zur Hausen, A., Gitsch, G., and Stickeler, E., 2005, Specific induction of pp125 focal adhesion kinase in human breast cancer, Brit. J. Cancer Aug 23; [Epub ahead of print].
78. Kim, S.J., Park, J.W., Yoon, J.S., Mok, J.O., Kim, Y.J., Park, H.K., Kim, C.H., Byun, D.W., Lee, Y.J., Jin, S.Y., Suh, K.I., and Yoo, M.H., 2004, Increased expression of focal adhesion kinase in thyroid cancer: immunohistochemical study, J. Korean Med. Sci. 19:710-715.
79. Grisaru-Granovsky, S., Salah, Z., Maoz, M., Pruss, D., Beller, U., and Bar-Shavit, R., 2005, Differential expression of protease activated receptor 1 (Par1) and pY397FAK in benign and malignant human ovarian tissue samples, Int. J. Cancer 113:372-378.
80. Gutenberg, A., Bruck, W., Buchfelder, M., and Ludwig, H.C., 2004, Expression of tyrosine kinases FAK and Pyk2 in 331 human astrocytomas, Acta Neuropathol. (Berl) 108:224-230.
81. Tamagiku, Y., Sonoda, Y., Kunisawa, M., Ichikawa, D., Murakami, Y., Aizu-Yokota, E., and Kasahara, T., 2004, Down-regulation of procaspase-8 expression by focal adhesion kinase protects HL-60 cells from TRAIL-induced apoptosis, Biochem. Biophys. Res. Commun. 323:445-452.
82. Beinke, C., van Beuningen, D., and Cordes, N., 2003, Ionizing radiation modulates expression and tyrosine phosphorylation of the focal adhesion-associated proteins focal adhesion kinase (FAK) and its substrates p130cas and paxillin in A549 human lung carcinoma cells in vitro, Int. J. Radiat. Biol. 79:721-731.
83. Riley, P.A., 1994, Free radicals in biology: oxidative stress and the effects of ionizing radiation, Int. J. Radiat. Biol. 65:27-33.
84. Zent, R., Ailenberg, M., Downey, GP., and Silverman, M., 1999, ROS stimulate reorganization of mesangial cell-collagen gels by tyrosine kinase signaling, Am. J. Physiol. 276:F278-87.
85. Riedl, S.J., and Shi, Y., 2004, Molecular mechanisms of caspase regulation during apoptosis, Nat. Rev. Mol. Cell Biol. 5:897-907.
86. Sastry, S.K., and Burridge, K., 2000, Focal adhesions: a nexus for intracellular signaling and cytoskeletal dynamics, Exp Cell Res. 261:25-36.
87. Hsu, S.L., Cheng, C.C., Shi, Y.R., and Chiang, C.W., 2001, Proteolysis of integrin alpha5 and beta1 subunits involved in retinoic acid-induced apoptosis in human hepatoma Hep3B cells, Cancer Lett. 167:193-204.
88. Adams, S.W., Wang, L., Fortney, J., and Gibson, L.F., 2004, Etoposide differentially affects bone marrow and dermal derived endothelial cells, J. Cell Mol. Med. 8:338-348.
89. Utsubo, R., Sonoda, Y., Takahashi, R., Iijima, S., Aizu-Yokota, E., and Kasahara, T., 2004, Proteome analysis of focal adhesion kinase (FAK)-overexpressing cells, Biol. Pharm. Bull. 27:1735-1741.
90. Persad, S., Attwell, S., Gray, V., Delcommenne, M., Troussard, A., Sanghera, J., and Dedhar, S., 2000, Inhibition of integrin-linked kinase (ILK) suppresses activation of

protein kinase B/Akt and induces cell cycle arrest and apoptosis of PTEN-mutant prostate cancer cells, Proc. Natl. Acad. Sci. USA 97:3207–3212.
91. Takanami, I., 2005, Increased expression of integrin-linked kinase is associated with shorter survival in non-small cell lung cancer, BMC Cancer 5:1.
92. Bravou, V., Klironomos, G., Papadaki, E., Stefanou, D., and Varakis, J., 2003, Integrin-linked kinase (ILK) expression in human colon cancer, Brit. J. Cancer 89:2340-2341.
93. Ito, R., Oue, N., Zhu, X., Yoshida, K., Nakayama, H., Yokozaki, H., and Yasui, W., 2003, Expression of integrin-linked kinase is closely correlated with invasion and metastasis of gastric carcinoma, Virchows Arch. 442:118-123.
94. Ahmed, N., Riley, C., Oliva, K., Stutt, E., Rice, G.E., and Quinn, M.A., 2003, Integrin-linked kinase expression increases with ovarian tumour grade and is sustained by peritoneal tumour fluid, J. Pathol. 201:229-237.
95. Dai, D.L., Makretsov, N., Campos, E.I., Huang, C., Zhou, Y., Huntsman, D., Martinka, M., and Li, G., 2003, Increased expression of integrin-linked kinase is correlated with melanoma progression and poor patient survival, Clin. Cancer Res. 9:4409-4414.
96. Delcommenne, M., Tan, C., Gray, V., Ruel, L., Woodgett, J., and Dedhar, S., 1998, Phosphoinositide-3-OH kinase-dependent regulation of glycogen synthase kinase 3 and protein kinase B/Akt by the integrin-linked kinase, Proc. Natl. Acad. Sci. USA 95:11211-11216.
97. Persad, S., Attwell, S., Gray, V., Mawji, N., Deng, J.T., Leung, D., Yan, J., Sanghera, J., Walsh, M.P., and Dedhar, S., 2001, Regulation of protein kinase B/Akt-serine 473 phosphorylation by integrin-linked kinase: critical roles for kinase activity and amino acids arginine 211 and serine 343, J. Biol. Chem. 276:27462-27469.
98. Attwell, S., Roskelley, C., and Dedhar, S., 2000, The integrin-linked kinase (ILK) suppresses anoikis, Oncogene 19:3811-3815.
99. Rearden, A., 1994, A new LIM protein containing an autoepitope homologous to "senescent cell antigen", Biochem. Biophys. Res. Commun. 201:1124-1131.
100. Wu, C., and Dedhar, S., 2001, Integrin-linked kinase (ILK) and its interactors: a new paradigm for the coupling of extracellular matrix to actin cytoskeleton and signaling complexes, J. Cell Biol. 155:505-510.
101. Duxbury, M.S., Ito, H., Benoit, E., Waseem, T., Ashley, S.W., and Whang, E.E., 2005, RNA interference demonstrates a novel role for integrin-linked kinase as a determinant of pancreatic adenocarcinoma cell gemcitabine chemoresistance, Clin. Cancer Res. 11:3433-3438.
102. Hannigan, G., Troussard, A.A., and Dedhar, S., 2005, Integrin-linked kinase: a cancer therapeutic target unique among its ILK, Nat. Rev. Cancer 5:51-63.
103. Edwards, L.A., Thiessen, B., Dragowska, W.H., Daynard, T., Bally, M.B., and Dedhar, S., 2005, Inhibition of ILK in PTEN-mutant human glioblastomas inhibits PKB/Akt activation, induces apoptosis, and delays tumor growth, Oncogene 24:3596-3605.
104. Yau, C.Y., Wheeler, J.J., Sutton, K.L., and Hedley, D.W., 2005, Inhibition of integrin-linked kinase by a selective small molecule inhibitor, QLT0254, inhibits the PI3K/PKB/mTOR, Stat3, and FKHR pathways and tumor growth, and enhances gemcitabine-induced apoptosis in human orthotopic primary pancreatic cancer xenografts, Cancer Res. 65:1497-504.
105. Tucker, G.C., 2002, Inhibitors of integrins, Curr. Opin. Pharmacol. 2:394-402.
106. Mousa, S.A., 2002, Anti-integrin as novel drug-discovery targets: Potential therapeutic ad diagnostic implications, Curr. Opin. Chem. Biol. 6:534-541.
107. Damiano, J.S., 2002, Integrins as novel drug targets for overcoming innate drug resistance, Curr. Cancer Drug Targets 2:37-43.

108. Rust, W.L., Carper, S.W., and Plopper, G.E., 2002, The promise of integrins as effective targets for anticancer agents, J. Biomed. Biotechnol. 2:124-130.
109. Tucker, G.C., 2003, Alpha v integrin inhibitors and cancer therapy, Curr. Opin. Investig. Drugs 4:722-731.
110. Hynes, N.E., and Lane, H.A., 2005, ERBB receptors and cancer: the complexity of targeted inhibitors, Nat. Rev. Cancer 5:341-354.
111. Baker, E.K., and El-Osta, A., 2003, The rise of DNA methylation and the importance of chromatin on multidrug resistance in cancer, Exp. Cell Res. 290:177-194.
112. Nardi, V., Azam, M., and Daley, G.Q., 2004, Mechanisms and implications of imatinib resistance mutations in BCR-ABL, Curr. Opin. Hematol. 11:35-43.

Chapter 9

CAM-DR: HANGING ON FOR CELL SURVIVAL

Lori A. Hazlehurst
Experimental Therapeutics Section, H. Lee Moffitt Cancer Center, Tampa, Florida, USA

Abstract: β1 integrin is known to be an important mediator of cell cycle kinetics, survival and differentiation. More recently evidence is accumulating that β1 integrin-mediated adhesion is sufficient to cause resistance to mechanistically distinct cytotoxics. This drug resistant phenotype is commonly referred to as **c**ell adhesion **m**ediated **d**rug **r**esistance or CAM-DR. The CAM-DR phenotype is observed in multiple tumor types that express a diverse array of oncogenes, suggesting that underlying resistant mechanism(s) do not require the expression of a specific oncogene for conferring the drug resistant phenotype. Despite the consistency of the drug resistant phenotype a single CAM-DR pathway has yet to emerge. However, current data suggest that alterations in cell cycle checkpoints and Bcl-2 family members are likely to be critical for conferring the CAM-DR phenotype. This chapter will discuss CAM-DR models and potential targets downstream of β1 integrin ligation that contribute to the drug resistant phenotype.

Key words: CAM-DR; β1 integrin; Bcl-2; Bim; drug resistance; cell cycle; β1 integrin splice variants

1. INTRODUCTION

The emergence of drug resistance continues to impede the success of chemotherapy. Resistance to chemotherapy can occur as a result of chronic drug exposure (acquired drug resistance) or by intrinsic mechanisms such as soluble or matrix induced activation of survival signals (de novo resistance). Acquired drug resistance models have been instrumental in elucidating drug resistant targets and in some cases have aided in the identification of drug targets (1, 2). These unicellular models have demonstrated that typically multiple mechanisms of resistance emerge following drug selection (3). Mechanisms that contribute to acquired drug resistance include decreased

A.E. Cress and R.B. Nagle (eds.), Cell Adhesion and Cytoskeletal Molecules in Metastasis, 163–177.

drug uptake, increased drug efflux, altered drug target, drug metabolism, alterations in DNA repair and cell cycle checkpoint pathways and changes in downstream mediators of the apoptotic pathway. The multi-factorial nature of acquired drug resistance makes therapeutic intervention a pharmacological challenge. In contrast, de novo resistance does not require drug selection for the expression of the resistant phenotype. The first selection pressure for the growth and maintenance of a tumor is the microenvironment, and thus it is likely that tumor progression results in the selection of cells that are efficient at utilizing survival signals generated in the microenvironment. These same survival signals that originate from host-tumor cell interactions can potentially contribute to de novo drug resistance. Sources of de novo resistance include signals that can be either paracrine or autocrine in nature.

Cell adhesion represents one potential signal that may contribute to de novo drug resistance. Detachment of many types of cells from the extracellular matrix can trigger apoptosis. This phenomena is referred to as anoikis, which is derived from the Greek word for "homelessness" (4). Anoikis is thought to represent an important mechanism for tissue maintenance and homeostasis. Resistance to anoikis is believed to be essential for tumor progression and metastasis to occur and, expression of certain oncogenes is known to confer resistance to anoikis induced cell death (5). We propose that although tumor cells are resistant to detachment induced cell death, that integrin activation continues to favor cell survival following cytotoxic insult even in anoikis resistant tumor cells. This suggests that resistance to anoikis does not result in the activation of a redundant integrin mediated pathway(s) but rather a complementary anti-apoptotic pathway. Results to support this include observations that adhesion of anchorage independent solid tumor cell lines via β1 integrins confers drug resistance. In addition, hematopoietic malignant cells are inherently resistant to anoikis mediated cell death, yet β1 integrin-mediated adhesion will confer resistance to cell death induced by cytotoxic insult. The following section will discuss potential mechanisms that are likely to contribute to drug resistance associated with β1 integrin mediated cell adhesion.

2. CAM-DR

Traditionally drug resistance mechanisms have been identified and functionally characterized in resistant cell lines developed by chronic exposure to a cytotoxic agent. However, these unicellular drug resistant models lack consideration of host-tumor cell interactions that may participate in the emergence of the drug resistant phenotype (see Figure 1).

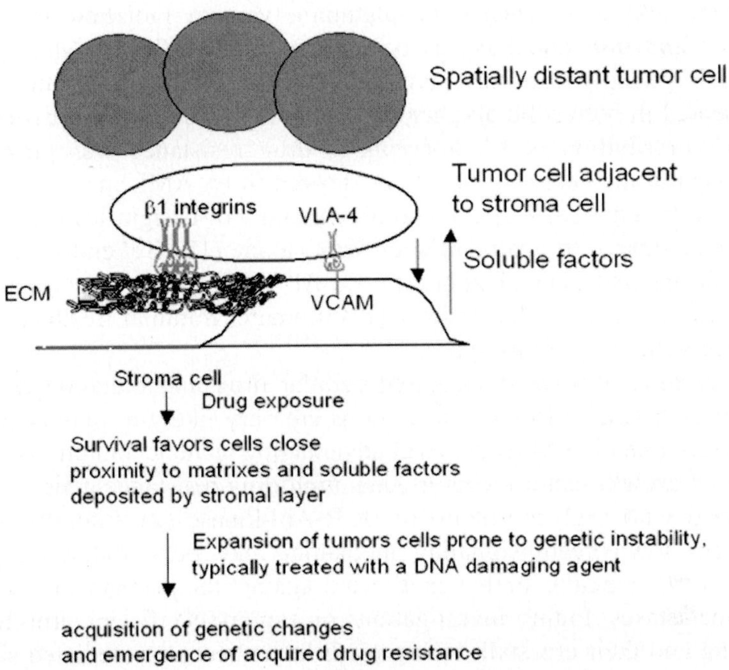

Figure 1. Proposed model of Cell Adhesion Mediated Drug Resistance (CAM-DR). Host tumor cell interactions participate in the emergence of the drug resistant phenotype. The tumor cell contains adhesion receptors such as the β1 integrin containing receptors (β1 integrins) or more specifically integrin α4β1 (VLA-4).

The first model demonstrating the effects of cell adhesion on drug resistance was reported by Durand and Sutherland in 1972 (7). These investigators demonstrated that V79 Chinese hamster cells grown as a spheroid culture was sufficient to cause radiation resistance relative to cells treated as a monolayer. These data suggest that cell-cell contact enhances survival of tumor cells in response to cytotoxic stimuli. However, this model did not identify the cell adhesion molecule(s) conferring the drug resistance phenotype. More recently several investigators have convincingly demonstrated that adhesion of cells in a monolayer culture via β1 integrins is sufficient to confer a multi-drug resistance phenotype (8-13). This phenotype is commonly referred to as cell adhesion mediated drug resistance or CAM-DR (14). The identification of an adhesion moiety that confers drug resistance has provided a good model for investigators to mechanistically dissect integrin-mediated pathways that confer drug resistance. The CAM-DR phenotype is characterized as a multi-drug drug resistant phenotype as resistance to mechanistically diverse cytotoxics including topoisomerase II inhibitors, alkylating agents, cis-platinum, gamma radiation, the Bcr-abl inhibitor **imatinib** and Fas has been demonstrated (8-16). Moreover, the CAM-DR phenotype occurs across divergent genetic backgrounds and is documented in both solid and hematopoietic malignancies. Validation of the *in vivo* contribution of β1 integrins to drug resistance was provided by Matsunaga et al. These investigators showed in an AML mouse model that treatment with a VLA-4 specific antibody and Ara-C significantly increased survival compared to treatment with Ara-C alone (17). Taken together, these data indicate that cellular adhesion via β1 integrins may contribute to de novo resistance and the failure to eliminate minimal residual disease observed with many tumor types.

Concerning existent or acquired cellular drug and radiation resistance, integrin-mediated cell-ECM interactions are very likely to play an essential role in combination with survival-advantaging genetic mutations in, e.g., epidermal growth factor receptor gene, multidrug resistance gene 1 (MDR1; associated with p-glycoprotein) or BCR-Abl-kinase (2). Integrin receptors and their downstream signaling mediators may be effective targets for innovative therapeutic strategies directed against the primary tumor as well as its metastases. Future investigations on tumor-specific integrin-mediated signaling and their crosstalk with growth factor receptor-mediated signaling may also substantially contribute to the identification of new molecular targets and the development of interacting substances for adjuvant chemo- and radiotherapy strategies.

It is likely that mediators of de novo resistance may also contribute to the emergence of acquired drug resistance. Teicher et al. were the first to demonstrate the influence of the tumor microenvironment in mediating the acquisition of drug resistance associated with chronic exposure to a cytotoxin (18). These investigators showed that treatment of mice bearing EMT-6 mammary tumors over a six-month period with alkylating agents resulted in the selection of a drug resistance phenotype that could be detected *in vivo*, but not in a unicellular tissue culture system. These studies were the first to show that components of the tumor microenvironment are required for the expression of a functional acquired drug resistance phenotype. More recent data has suggested that tumor cells may in fact remodel or condition the microenvironment to favor cell survival following insult by chemotherapeutic drugs. Sherman–Baust et al. showed that cisplatin resistant cells overexpressed collagen VI, and furthermore plates coated with collagen VI conferred platinum resistance to the parental A2780 drug sensitive ovarian cancer cell line (19). In addition, these investigators demonstrated in clinical specimens that strong collagen VI staining occurred only on the border between tumor and stromal cells. These results suggest that either tumor cells were directly depositing the matrix or that tumor cells stimulate adjacent stromal cells to deposit collagen V1. Moreover, our laboratory recently showed that cell adhesion via β1 integrins of U937 cells influences the acquisition of mitoxantrone resistance. In this study we directly compared the emerging drug resistant phenotype when cells were selected with mitoxantrone in a traditional suspension culture versus adherent to fibroenctin via β1 inetgrins. In comparing the phenotype we showed that both acquired drug resistant models demonstrated reduced drug induced DNA damage and a reduction in the drug target topoisomerase II. However, the mechanisms regulating topoisomerase II levels were divergent depending on the culture conditions. Cells selected in suspension showed reduced topoisomerase II protein levels, a finding that correlated with reduced mRNA levels. In contrast, chronic selection with mitoxantrone in adherent U937 cells resulted in post-transcriptional regulation of topoisomerase II (20). Together these data indicate that drug resistant models that recapitulate tumor-host interactions may be needed for the identification of clinically relevant de novo and acquired drug resistant targets.

Integrins do not contain intrinsic kinase activity, suggesting that cellular hardware could dictate response to integrin activation. In fact the response of β1 integrin, activation of downstream signaling events is often cell context specific. In addition, another dimension of complexity associated with integrin signaling is the potential crosstalk between cytokine and growth factor receptors. For example, in breast epithelial cells adhesion via α6β1 in the presence of insulin resulted in increased phosphorylation of the insulin receptor and protein kinase B (21). Despite dependency on downstream components and perhaps even cross talk with specific receptors contributing to diversity of integrin mediated signaling, the CAM-DR phenotype is observed across diverse genetic backgrounds with varied expression of oncogenes. For example, Bcr-abl expression is known to confer drug resistance, yet adhesion of Bcr-abl positive chronic myelogenous leukemia (CML) cell lines via β1 integrins confers an additional increase in drug resistance compared to CML cell lines treated in suspension cultures(14, 16). The challenge will be to determine whether the anti-apoptotic phenotype observed with β1 integrin mediated adhesion is the result of a consistent, but to date identified pathway(s), or rather if β1 integrins utilize divergent cellular hardware to confer a very similar CAM-DR phenotype.

3. TARGETS ASSOCIATED WITH CAM-DR

Although the signaling network mediating the CAM-DR phenotype is currently not well delineated, several downstream drug resistance targets have been identified as potential mediators of the CAM-DR phenotype.

These potential targets include BCL-2 family members, p27kip1, alterations in chromatin structure and topoisomerase II. The potential role of these targets will be further discussed in this chapter.

3.1 B.2. BCL-2 Family Members

Several reports have indicated that the levels of Bcl-2 family members are altered upon β1 inetgrin activation(22, 25). Bcl-2 family members can be sub-divided into two main categories. The anti-apoptotic group consists of Bcl-2, Bcl-xl, Mcl-1. These proteins contain 4 BH domains and promote cell survival by binding pro-apoptotic Bcl-2 family members and inhibiting their function. The proapoptotic Bcl-2 family can be further separated into two classes the multi BH domain proteins consisting of Bax and Bak and the BH3 only proteins consisting of Bmf, Bid, Bim, Bad, Bik, Puma and Noxa.

The BH3 pro-apoptotic member, Bim has recently emerged as a potential mediator of the CAM-DR phenotype in hematopoietic malignant tumor cells. Bim knockout studies have revealed that Bim is an important regulator of leukocyte homeostasis, as $Bim^{-/-}$ mice show accumulation of B cells, mature T-cells, granulocytes and monocytes compared to wild type mice (26). Furthermore, B-cells derived from $Bim^{-/-}$ mice were resistant to spontaneous induced apoptosis as well as gamma radiation, ionomycin and dexamethasone induced cell death. To date 10 Bim splice variants have been reported in genebank. Bim_{EL} is the most highly expressed isoform and can be easily identified by molecular weight by separation on a one dimensional SDS-PAGE. Bim_{EL} contains the Erk1/2 phosphoryaltion site, the dynein motor binding site and a hydrophobic domain (see Figure 2). Bim_L and Bim_S represent two other splice variants that are most commonly reported as being expressed in tumor cells in the literature, however, it must be cautioned that these two smaller isoforms are more difficult to identify based solely on molecule weight. Both Bim_{EL} and Bim_L contain the dynein motor binding motif, JNK phosphorylation site and the hydrophobic domain (27). Transfection studies have shown that Bim_S is the most potent inducer of apoptosis and lacks the dynein binding motif but does contain the hydrophobic domain required for mitochondria targeting (28).

Bim protein levels were decreased when hematopoietic tumor cell lines were adhered to fibronectin via β1 integrins (25). Current understanding suggests that Bim is tightly regulated by multiple mechanisms including localization, transcriptional regulation and by proteasome mediated degradation. Investigations have shown that activation of the MAPK signaling pathway promotes phosphorylation and proteasome dependent degradation of Bim_{EL} (29). In addition, to Erk1/2 regulation of Bim protein levels, c-Cbl has been implicated in regulating Bim protein levels. Recently

Akiyama et al., showed a physical interaction of c-Cbl and Bim (30). Moreover, these same investigators showed that osteoclasts derived from a c-Cbl-/- mice failed to reduce Bim levels when stimulated with M-CSF compared to wild type cells. Together, these data indicate that c-Cbl may be an important regulator of Bim degradation. c-Cbl has multiple functions both as an adaptor protein and an E3 ligase. Furthermore c-Cbl is known to bind both paxillin and tubulin, and can be found in focal adhesion complexes (31, 32). Further studies are warranted to determine whether c-Cbl plays a role in β1 integrin mediated attenuation of Bim protein levels.

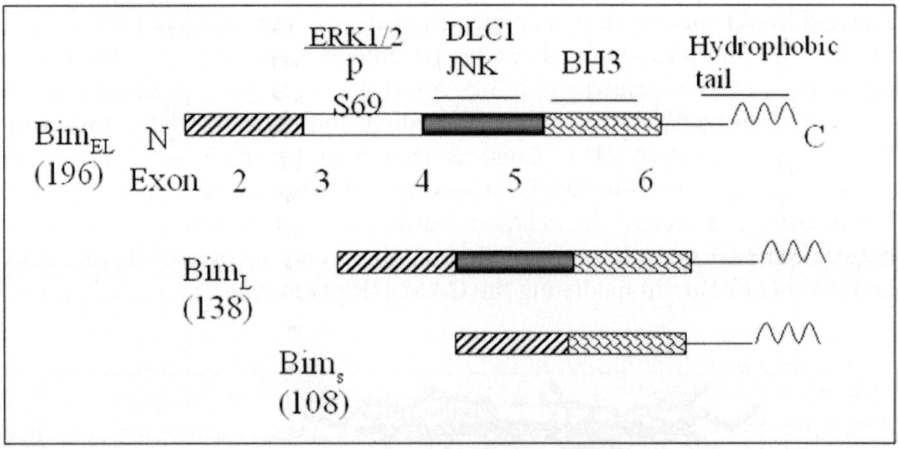

Figure 2. Bim splice variants. Only Bim$_{el}$ contains the ERK1/2 phosporylation site. Bim$_{el}$ and Bim$_L$ contain the dyenin motor complex domain and JNK phosphorylation site. All three splice variants contain one BH3 domain and a hydrophobic tail required for targeting to the mitochonria membrane.

Trafficking of Bim is another mode of Bim regulation. Puthalakath et al. initially reported that the dynein motor complex sequesters Bim in healthy cells (33). This was supported by evidence showing that Bim is bound to the LC8 component of the microtubule. In addition these same investigators showed that following cytotoxic insult LC8 and Bim was trafficked from the dynein motor complex to the mitochondria membrane were Bim was found to be bound to Bcl-2. In contrast, Zhu et al. showed that in healthy T-cells Bim was bound to either Bcl-xl or BCL-2 in the mitochondria (34). Thus the localization of Bim in healthy cells may be context specific. There is some evidence that JNK dependent phosphorylation of Bim$_L$ following cytotoxic insult may release Bim$_L$ from the dynein motor complex (27). However, again this maybe cell context specific because Puthalakath et al., showed that following apoptotic stimuli Bim_L was trafficked to the mitochondria via DLC1.

Transcriptional regulation of Bim appears to be predominately driven by Foxo3a. The promoter region of Bim contains a Forkhead responsive element and ChIP assays have determined that Foxo3a binds to the promoter region of Bim (35). Phosphorylation of Foxo3a results in cytoplasmic localization of Foxo3a and thereby inhibits the transcriptional function of the protein. SGK1 and Akt share similar consensus phosphorylation sites (RXTXXS/T). However, recently Brunet et al., showed for the substrate Foxo3a, that SGK1 had a preference for Ser-315 while Akt phosphorylated Ser-253 more efficiently compared to SGK1(36). These data suggests that Akt and SGK1 may work in a cooperative rather than redundant fashion with respects to phosphorylating Foxo3a. β1 Integrin activation is reported to activate the MAPK pathway (37, 38), AKT(39), SGK1(40). In addition c-cbl is a known to be recruited to focal adhesions and phosphorylated following β1 integrin activation (41). Thus, as shown in Figure 3, integrins could potentially regulate Bim levels at multiple levels including transcription, localization and protein degradation. Further studies are warranted to better delineate the β1 integrin pathway that regulates Bim levels in adherent cells and the role of Bim in mediating the CAM-DR phenotype.

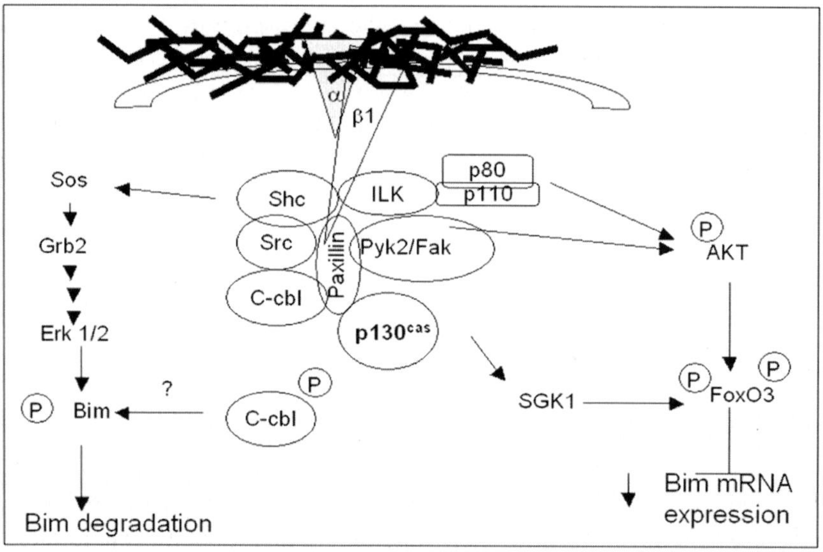

Figure 3. Candidate downstream signaling cascades involved in CAM-DR involving Bim regulation. Two arms of the signaling cascades are envisioned to either impact the suppression of Bim mRNA expression or the increase in Bim degradation.

3.2 Effects on Cell Cycle

The potency of many anti-cancer agents that cause DNA damage is often reduced in quiescent cells. (42-44). Experimental evidence to support this concept includes reports where the ectopic expression of either the CDK2 inhibitor p21 or $p27^{Kip1}$ is causative for resistance to DNA damaging drugs (43, 44). Thus, signals that cause reversible growth arrest in tumor cells could transiently protect from apoptosis induced by DNA damaging agents. The effects of integrin-mediated adhesion on cell cycle appear to be cell context specific. The divergent effect on cell cycle progression of β1 integrin mediated adhesion is most likely the result of the relative abundance of β1-integrin splice variants and not due to differences in cellular hardware. Four naturally occurring splice variants of the β1 integrin have been identified, and the splicing occurs within the cytoplasmic domain of each β1 integrin variant (45). These four β1 integrin splice variants are designated β1A, β1B, β1C and β1D, and evidence shows that activation of specific splice variants results in divergent signal transduction pathways. For example, activation of the β1A integrin splice variant is associated with activation of the MAPK pathway and cell cycle progression (46) (37, 47). In contrast, activation of either the β1D or β1C integrin splice variant is associated with the inhibition of cell cycle progression (48, 49). While, the activation of β1B appears to act as a dominant negative, and inhibits cellular adhesion and motility (50). Evidence also exists demonstrating that the expression of β1-integrin splice variants is different depending on the tissue type. For example, the β1A splice variant is the most ubiquitously expressed β1 integrin variant while the β1C splice variant is known to be expressed in epithelial cells of the liver, placenta, platelets as well as monocytic and erthroleukemia cell lines but is not expressed in peripheral blood lymphocytes (51). In contrast, the β1D isoform has only been detected in striated muscle cells (52). Recently, Fornaro et al. demonstrated that transfection of β1C in CHO-K1 cells caused an increase in $p27^{Kip1}$ protein levels, and furthermore decreasing $p27^{Kip1}$ levels by $p27^{Kip1}$ antisense treatment abrogated the inhibitory effects of β1C on DNA synthesis (53). In summary, the majority of data indicates that the diverse effect of β1 integrin mediated adhesion on cell cycle kinetics is due to the relative expression of β1 integrin splice variants rather than differences in downstream signaling complexes.

Adhesion of normal CD34+ cells to fibronectin is reported to both inhibit spontaneous apoptosis and induce growth arrest (54-56). In addition, prolonged adhesion of a multiple myeloma cell line to fibronectin resulted in a reversible cell cycle arrest at the G1/S boundary. This observation correlated with increased $p27^{Kip1}$ levels and inhibition of CDK2 kinase activity. Moreover, reducing $p27^{Kip1}$ levels by antisense treatment increased etoposide induced apoptosis in adherent cells (9). In addition, to integrin mediated effects on basal cell cycle effects, β1 integrin mediated cell adhesion has been reported to increase percentages of cells blocked in G2/M following radiation treatment. Binding of human lung cancer cell line to fibronectin via β1 inetgrins resulted in increased G2/M block and resistance to gamma radiation. (13). Similarly, adhesion of normal breast and prostate cell lines to laminin 5 via α6β4 enhanced the radiation dependent G2/M block. However in this context activation of α6β4 did not alter cell survival (57). This may reflect differences in either the ability of β integrins to confer resistance to cytotoxics or differences in transformed versus normal cells in response to integrin ligation.

3.3 Chromatin Structure and DNA Damage

Integrin engagement is most often studied in the context of immediate signaling originating at the focal adhesion contacts. However, it is becoming clear that not only does integrin binding result in changes in cytoskeletal and plasma membrane structure at the leading edge but also causes dramatic changes in nuclear structure. Jones et al. showed that β1 integrin mediated engagement of endothelial cells results in increased sensitivity to microccocal nuclease digestion, suggesting that the chromatin of adherent cells is more relaxed compared to cells cultured in suspension (58). This same group more recently showed that integrin engagement of endothelial cells results in increased acetylation of histone H3 (59). We have observed a similar finding as U937 cells adherent to fibronectin are more sensitive to Dnase I digestion (unpublished data) compared to cells cultured in suspension. In addition, pre-adhesion of U937 resulted in alterations in the nuclear pool of the drug target topoisomerase IIβ in adherent cells. Alterations in the nuclear pool of topoisomerase IIβ was shown by confocal microscopy and by finding that topoisomerase IIβ was resistant to salt extraction in nuclear extracts prepared from adherent cells compared to suspension cultures. Topoisomerase IIβ has been shown to bind to components of the NuRD chromatin remodeling complex, including HDAC1, HDAC2 and MTA (metastasis-associated tumor protein) (60). It is feasible although to date no experimental evidence exits that nuclear remodeling is essential for nuclear movement that occurs during cell polarization and migration. It is well known that metastastic tumor cells are resistant to chemotherapy, what is not known is whether drug resistance is due to genetic changes, the new environment or rather if the process of migration is sufficient to confer the drug resistant phenotype.

4. SUMMARY

Adhesion of both hematopoietic malignant and solid tumors via β1 integrins to components of the extracellular matrix is sufficient to confer resistance to mechanistically distinct cytotoxics. β1 integrin-mediated adhesion has emerged as a viable target to increase the efficacy of currently uses cytotoxics. The target has been validated in both animal models and primary malignant specimens (61, 25). Thus the culmination of evidence suggests that β1 integrin-mediated adhesion is likely to have clinical relevance and may contribute to the failure to eliminate minimal residual disease. Several putative targets have been identified including changes in cell cycle checkpoints and alterations in the level of expression of pro and anti-apoptotic Bcl-2 family members. Further studies are needed to determine whether blocking β1 integrin mediated adhesion or downstream signaling will be the best approach for inhibiting CAM-DR and improving the efficacy of currently used cytotoxics.

REFERENCES

1. Dalton, W.S. and Salmon, S.E. Drug resistance in myeloma: mechanisms and approaches to circumvention. Hematol. Oncol. Clin. North Am., 6: 383-393, 1992.
2. Gottesman, M.M., Fojo, T., and Bates, S.E. Multidrug resistance in cancer: role of ATP-dependent transporters. Nat.Rev. Cancer, 2: 48-58, 2002.
3. Hazlehurst, L.A., Foley, N.E., Gleason-Guzman, M.C., Hacker, M.P., Cress A.E., Greenberger, L.W., De Jong, M.C., and Dalton, W.S. Multiple mechanisms confer drug-resistance to mitoxantrone in the human 8226 myeloma cll line. Cancer Research, 59: 1021-1028, 1999.
4. Frisch, S.M. and Francis, H. Disruption of epithelial cell-matrix interactions induces apoptosis. J. Cell Biol., 124: 619-626, 1994.
5. Windham, T.C., Parikh, N.U., Siwak, D.R., Summy, J.M., McConkey, D.J., Kraker, A.J., and Gallick, G.E. Src activation regulates anoikis in human colon tumor cell lines. Oncogene, 21: 7797-7807, 2002.
6. Rosen, K., Rak, J., Leung, T., Dean, N.M., Kerbel, R.S., and Filmus, J. Activated Ras prevents downregulation of Bcl-X(L) triggered by detachment from the extracellular matrix. A mechanism of Ras-induced resistance to anoikis in intestinal epithelial cells. J.Cell Biol., 149: 447-456, 2000.
7. Durand, R.E. and Sutherland, R.M. Effects of intercellular contact on repair of radiation damage. Experimental Cell Research, 71: 75-80, 1972.
8. Damiano, J.S., Cress, A.E., Hazlehurst, L.A., Shtil, A.A., and Dalton, W.S. Cell adhesion mediated drug resistance (CAM-DR): Role of integrins and resistance to apoptosis in human myeloma cell lines. Blood, 93: 1658-1667, 1999.
9. Hazlehurst, L.A., Damiano J.S., BuyuksalmI., Pledger W.J., and Dalton W.S. Adhesion to fibronectin regulates p27kip1 levels and contributes to cell adhesion mediated drug resistance (CAM-DR). Oncogene, 38: 4319-4327, 2000.

10. Hazlehurst, L.A., Valkov, N., Wisner, L., Storey, J.A., Boulware, D., Sullivan, D.M., and Dalton, W.S. Reduction in drug-induced DNA double strand-breaks associated with β1 integrin-mediated adhesion correlates with drug resistance in U937 cells. Blood, 98: 1897-1903, 2001.
11. Sethi, T., Rintoul, R.C., Moore, S.M., MacKinnon, A.C., Salter, D., Choo, C., Chilvers E.R., Dransfield, I., Donnelly, S.C., Streiter, R., and Haslett, C. Extracellular matrix proteins protect small cell lung cancer cells against apoptosis: A mechanism for small cell lung cancer growth and drug resistance in vivo. Nature Medicine, 5: 662-668, 1999.
12. Aoudjit, F. and Vuori, K. Integrin signaling inhibits paclitaxel-induced apoptosis in breast cancer cells. Oncogene, 20: 4995-5004, 2001.
13. Cordes, N. and van Beuningen, D. Arrest of human lung fibroblasts in G2 phase after irradiation is regulated by converging phosphatidylinositol-3 kinase and beta1-integrin signaling in vitro. Int. J. Radiat. Oncol. Biol. Phys., 58: 453-462, 2004.
14. Damiano, J.S., Hazlehurst, L.A., and Dalton, W.S. Cell adhesion mediated resistance (CAM-DR) protects the K562 chronic myelogenous leukemia cell line from apoptosis induced by BCR/ABL inhibition cyctoxic drugs and γ radiation. Leukemia, 15: 1232-1239, 2001.
15. Shain, K.H., Landowski, T.H., and Dalton, W.S. Adhesion-mediated intracellular redistribution of c-Fas-associated death domain-like IL-1-converting enzyme-like inhibitory protein-long confers resistance to CD95-induced apoptosis in hematopoietic cancer cell lines. J.Immunol., 168: 2544-2553, 2002.
16. van der, K.H., Goetz, A.W., Miething, C., Duyster, J., and Aulitzky, W.E. Adhesion to fibronectin selectively protects Bcr-Abl+ cells from DNA damage-induced apoptosis. Blood, 98: 1532-1541, 2001.
17. Matsunaga, T., Takemoto, N., Sato, T., Takimoto, R., Tanaka, I., Fujimi, A., Akiyama, T., Kuroda, H., Kawano, Y., Kobune, M., Kato, J., Hirayama, Y., Sakamaki, S., Kohda, K., Miyake, K., and Niitsu, Y. Interaction between leukemic-cell VLA-4 and stromal fibronectin is a decisive factor for minimal residual disease of acute myelogenous leukemia. Nat. Med., 9: 1158-1165, 2003.
18. Teicher, B.A., Herman, T.S., Holden, S.A., Wang, Y.Y., Pfeffer, M.R., Crawford, J.W., and Frei, E.I. Tumor resistance to alkylating agents conferred by mechanisms operative only in vivo. Science, 247: 1457-1460, 1990.
19. Sherman-Baust, C.A., Weeraratna, A.T., Rangel, L.B., Pizer, E.S., Cho, K.R., Schwartz, D.R., Shock, T., and Morin, P.J. Remodeling of the extracellular matrix through overexpression of collagen VI contributes to cisplatin resistance in ovarian cancer cells. Cancer Cell, 3: 377-386, 2003.
20. Hazlehurst, L.A., Argilagos, R.F., Emmons, M., Boulware, D., Beam, C.A., Sullivan D.M. and Dalton, W.S. Cell Adhesion to fibronectin (CAM-DR) influences acquired mitoxantrone resistance in U937 cells. In Press Cancer Research, 2006.
21. Farrelly, N., Lee, Y.J., Oliver, J., Dive, C., and Streuli, C.H. Extracellular matrix regulates apoptosis in mammary epithelium through a control on insulin signaling. J. Cell Biol., 144: 1337-1348, 1999.
22. de la Fuente, M.T., Casanova, B., Moyano, J.V., Garcia-Gila, M., Sanz, L., Garcia-Marco, J., Silva, A., and Garcia-Pardo, A. Engagement of alpha4beta1 integrin by fibronectin induces in vitro resistance of B chronic lymphocytic leukemia cells to fludarabine. J. Leukoc. Biol., 71: 495-502, 2002.
23. Matter, M.L. and Ruoslahti, E.A signaling pathway from the alpha5beta1 and alpha(v)beta3 integrins that elevates bcl-2 transcription. J. Biol. Chem., 276: 27757-27763, 2001.

24. Gilmore, A.P., Metcalfe, A.D., Romer, L.H., and Streuli, C.H. Integrin-mediated survival signals regulate the apoptotic function of Bax through its conformation and subcellular localization. J. Cell Biol., 149: 431-446, 2000.
25. Hazlehurst, L.A., Enkemann, S., Beam, C., Argilagos, R.F., Painter, J., Shain, K., Saporta, S., Boulware, D., Mosciniski, M., Alsina, M., and Dalton, W.S. Genotypic and phenotypic comparisons of de novo and acquired melphalan resistance in an isogenic multiple myeloma cell line model. Cancer Research, 56: 660-670, 2003.
26. Bouillet, P., Metcalf, D., Huang, D.C., Tarlinton, D.M., Kay, T.W., Kontgen, F., Adams, J.M., and Strasser, A. Proapoptotic Bcl-2 relative Bim required for certain apoptotic responses, leukocyte homeostasis, and to preclude autoimmunity. Science, 286: 1735-1738, 1999.
27. Lei, K. and Davis, R.J. JNK phosphorylation of Bim-related members of the Bcl2 family induces Bax-dependent apoptosis. Proc. Natl. Acad. Sci. USA, 100: 2432-2437, 2003.
28. Marani, M., Tenev, T., Hancock, D., Downward, J., and Lemoine, N.R. Identification of novel isoforms of the BH3 domain protein Bim which directly activate Bax to trigger apoptosis. Mol. Cell Biol., 22: 3577-3589, 2002.
29. Ley, R., Balmanno, K., Hadfield, K., Weston, C., and Cook, S.J. Activation of the ERK1/2 signaling pathway promotes phosphorylation and proteasome-dependent degradation of the BH3-only protein, Bim. J. Biol. Chem., 278: 18811-18816, 2003.
30. Akiyama, T., Bouillet, P., Miyazaki, T., Kadono, Y., Chikuda, H., Chung, U.I., Fukuda, A., Hikita, A., Seto, H., Okada, T., Inaba, T., Sanjay, A., Baron, R., Kawaguchi, H., Oda, H., Nakamura, K., Strasser, A., and Tanaka, S. Regulation of osteoclast apoptosis by ubiquitylation of proapoptotic BH3-only Bcl-2 family member Bim. EMBO J., 22: 6653-6664, 2003.
31. Tsygankov, A.Y., Teckchandani, A.M., Feshchenko, E.A., and Swaminathan, G. Beyond the RING: CBL proteins as multivalent adapters. Oncogene, 20: 6382-6402, 2001.
32. Teckchandani, A.M., Birukova, A.A., Tar, K., Verin, A.D., and Tsygankov, A.Y. The multidomain protooncogenic protein c-Cbl binds to tubulin and stabilizes microtubules. Exp. Cell Res., 306: 114-127, 2005.
33. Puthalakath, H., Huang, D.C., O'Reilly, L.A., King, S.M., and Strasser, A. The proapoptotic activity of the Bcl-2 family member Bim is regulated by interaction with the dynein motor complex. Mol. Cell, 3: 287-296, 1999.
34. Zhu, Y., Swanson, B.J., Wang, M., Hildeman, D.A., Schaefer, B.C., Liu, X., Suzuki, H., Mihara, K., Kappler, J., and Marrack, P. Constitutive association of the proapoptotic protein Bim with Bcl-2-related proteins on mitochondria in T cells. Proc. Natl. Acad. Sci. USA, 101: 7681-7686, 2004.
35. Essafi, A., Fernandez, d.M., Hassen, Y.A., Soeiro, I., Mufti, G.J., Thomas, N.S., Medema, R.H., and Lam, E.W. Direct transcriptional regulation of Bim by FoxO3a mediates STI571-induced apoptosis in Bcr-Abl-expressing cells. Oncogene, 2005.
36. Brunet, A., Park, J., Tran, H., Hu, L.S., Hemmings, B.A., and Greenberg, M.E. Protein kinase SGK mediates survival signals by phosphorylating the forkhead transcription factor FKHRL1 (FOXO3a). Mol. Cell Biol., 21: 952-965, 2001.
37. Lin, T.H., Aplin, A.E., Shen, Y., Chen, Q., Schaller, M., Romer, L., Aukhil, I., and Juliano, R.L. Integrin-mediated activation of MAP kinase is independent of FAK:evidence for dual integrin signaling pathways in fibroblasts. Journal of Cell Biology, 136: 1385-1395, 1997.
38. Chen, Q., Lin, T.H., Der, C.J., and Juliano, R.L. Integrin-mediated activation of MEK and mitogen-activated protein kinase is independent of Ras [corrected]. J. Biol. Chem., 271: 18122-18127, 1996.

39. Lee J.W. and Juliano R.L. Alpha 5 beta 1 integrin protects intestinal epithelial cells from apoptosis through a phosphatidylinositol 3-kinase and protein kinase B-dependent pathway. Molecular Biology of the Cell, 11: 1973-1987, 2000.
40. Shelly, C. and Herrera, R. Activation of SGK1 by HGF, Rac1 and integrin-mediated cell adhesion in MDCK cells: PI-3K-dependent and -independent pathways. J. Cell Sci., 115: 1985-1993, 2002.
41. Manie, S.N., Sattler, M., Astier, A., Phifer, J.S., Canty, T., Morimoto, C., Druker, B.J., Salgia, R., Griffin, J.D., and Freedman, A.S. Tyrosine phosphorylation of the product of the c-cbl protooncogene is [corrected] induced after integrin stimulation. Exp. Hematol., 25: 45-50, 1997.
42. Solary, E., Bertrand R., Kohn, K.W., and Pommier, Y. Differential induction of apoptosis in undifferentiated and differentiated HL-60 cells by DNA toposiomerase I and II inhibitors. Blood, 81: 1359-1368, 1993.
43. Ruan, S., Okcu, F.M., Ren, J.P., Chiao, P., Andreeff, M., Levin, V., and Zhang, W. Overexpressed WAF1/CIP1 renders glioblastoma cells resistant to chemotherapy agents 1,3-Bis(2-chloroethyl)-1-nitrosurea and cisplatin. Cancer Research, 58: 1538-1543, 1998.
44. Eymin B., Haugg, M., Droin, N., Sordet, O., Dimanche-Boitrel, M.T., and Solary, E. p27Kip1 induces drug resistance by preventing apoptosis upstream of cytochrome c release and procaspase-3 activation in leukemic cells. Oncogene, 18: 1411-1418, 1999.
45. Fornaro, M. and Languino, L.R. Alternatively spliced variants:A new veiw of the integrin cytoplasmic domain. Matrix Biology, 16: 185-193, 1997.
46. Fornaro, M., Steger, C.A., Bennett, A.M., Wu, J.J., and Languino, L.R. Differential role of beta(1C) and beta(1A) integrin cytoplasmic variants in modulating focal adhesion kinase, protein kinase B/AKT, and Ras/Mitogen-activated protein kinase pathways. Mol.Biol.Cell, 11: 2235-2249, 2000.
47. Zhao, J.H., Reiske, H., and Guan, J.L. Regulation of the cell cycle by focal adhesion kinase. Journal of Cell Biology, 143: 1997-2008, 1997.
48. Belkin, A.M. and Retta, S.F. β_1D integrin inhibits cell cycle progression in normal myoblasts and fibroblasts. Journal of Biological Chemistry, 273: 15234-15240, 1998.
49. Meredith, J., Takada Y., Fornaro, M., Languino, L.R., and Schwartz, M.A. Inhibition of the cell cycle progression by the alternatively spliced integrin β_{1c}. Science, 269: 1570-1572, 1995.
50. Balzac, F., Retta, S.F., Albini, A., Melchiorri, A., Koteliansky, V.E., Geuna, M., Silengo, L., and Tarone, G. Expression of β1B integrin isoform in CHO cells results in a dominant negative effect on cell adhesion and motility. Journal Cell Biology, 127:557-565: 1994.
51. Languino, L. and Ruoslahti, E. An alternative form of the integrin β_1 subunit with a variant cytoplasmic domain. Journal of Biological Chemistry, 267 : 7116-7120, 1992.
52. Belkin, A.M., Zhidkova, N.I., Balzac, F., Altruda, F., Tomats, D., Maier, A., Tarone, G., Koteliansky, V.A., and Burridge, K. β1D integrin displaces the β1A isoform in striated muscles:Localization at junctional structures and signaling potential in nonmuscle cells. Journal Cell Biology, 132: 211-226, 1996.
53. Fornaro, M., Tallini, G., Zheng, D.Q., Flanagan, W.M., Manzotti, M., and Languino, L.R. p27(kip1) acts as a downstream effector of and is coexpressed with the beta1C integrin in prostatic adenocarcinoma. J. Clin. Invest, 103: 321-329, 1999.
54. Wang, M.W., Consoli, U., Lane, C.M., Durett, A., Lauppe, M.J., Champlin, R., Andreeff, M., and Deisseroth, A.B. Rescue from apoptosis in early (CD34-selected) versus late (non-CD34-selected) human hematopoietic cells by very late antigen 4- and

vascular cell adhesion molecule (VCAM) 1-dependent adhesion to bone marrow stromal cells. Cell Growth Differ., 9: 105-112, 1998.
55. Hurley, R.W., McCarthy, J.B., and Verfaille, C.M. Direct adhesion to bone marrow stroma via fibronectin receptors inhibits hematopoietic progenitor proliferation. Journal Clinical Investigations, 96: 511-519, 1995.
56. Hurley, R.W., McCarthy, J.B., Wayner, E.A., and Verfaille, C.M. Monoclonal antibody crosslinking of the α4 or β1 integrin inhibits committed clonogenic hematopoietic progenitor proliferation. Experimental Hematology, 25: 321-328, 1997.
57. Kremer, C.L., Schmelz, M., and Cress, A.E. Integrin-dependent amplification of the G2 arrest induced by ionizing radiation. Prostate, 2005.
58. Jones, C.B., McIntosh, J., Huang, H., Graytock, A., Hoyt, D.G. Regulation of bleomycin-induced DNA breakage and chromatin structure in lung endothelial cells by integrins and poly(ADP-ribose)polymerase. Mol Pharmacol. 59:69-75, 2001.
59. Rose, J.L., Huang, H., Wray, S.F., and Hoyt, D.G. Integrin engagement increases histone H3 acetylation and reduces histone H1 association with DNA in murine lung endothelial cells. Mol. Pharmacol., 68: 439-446, 2005.
60. Tsai, S., Valkov, N., Yang, W., Gunp, J., Sullivan, D., and Seto E. Histone deactylase interacts directly with DNA toposiomerase II. Nature Genetics, 26: 349-353, 2000.
61. Matsunaga, T., Takemoto, N., Sato, T., Takimoto, R., Tanaka, I., Fujimi, A., Akiyama, T., Kuroda, H., Kawano, Y., Kobune, M., Kato, J., Hirayama, Y., Sakamaki, S., Kohda, K., Miyake, K., and Niitsu, Y. Interaction between leukemic-cell VLA-4 and stromal fibronectin is a decisive factor for minimal residual disease of acute myelogenous leukemia. Nat. Med., 9: 1158-1165, 2003.

Chapter 10

EPITHELIAL CELL SURFACE TARGETING USING SYNTHETIC D-AMINO ACID PEPTIDES

Thomas C. Sroka[1], Anne E. Cress[1], and Kit S. Lam[2]
[1]Arizona Cancer Center, University of Arizona, Tucson, AZ, USA. [2]University of California Davis Cancer Center, Division of Hematology/Oncology and the Department of Internal Medicine, University of California, Davis, CA, USA

Abstract: The cell surface of epithelial cancers is known to change dramatically during tumor progression. The alteration of the cancer cell surface is distinct from the normal cell surface from which the cancer is derived and provides an attractive potential target for diagnostic, prognostic or therapeutic intervention. In recent years, it has been appreciated that while a vast majority of tumor cell surfaces become devoid of cell surface markers, a cohort of cell adhesion receptors are persistently expressed on tumor cells throughout the different stages of metastasis. In this chapter, we will focus on the use of combinatorial peptide chemistry techniques with biological approaches to isolate tumor cell adhesion d-amino acid peptides. These peptides when immobilized are capable of supporting tumor cell adhesion but block cell spreading and the downstream activation of focal adhesion kinase or mitogen activated kinase kinase. These results suggest that D-amino acid peptides can be discovered using a cell adhesion assay as a successful screen for bioactive peptides. Further, the immobilized peptides will uncouple cellular adhesion from the downstream signaling events. This strategy can select for cell adhesion peptides capable of both capturing cancer cells and blocking downstream signaling events.

Key words: peptides; cell surface; epithelial cancer; D-amino acid; signaling

1. INTRODUCTION

Most cancer deaths are directly from the consequences of metastatic tumors rather than the primary tumor itself (1, 2). There is a great need for new therapeutics to target the metastatic process given that cancer diagnosis often occurs at a relatively late stage in cancer progression. In order to

A.E. Cress and R.B. Nagle (eds.), Cell Adhesion and Cytoskeletal Molecules in Metastasis, 179–192.

develop novel therapeutics, further research is needed to identify the critical molecular components involved in metastasis. Although metastasis is a complicated *in vivo* process, it is valuable to initially examine the molecular components at the cellular level *in vitro*. In general, study of the machinery responsible for cellular motility can lead to the important discovery of key molecular players that regulate cell migration and/or invasion. Some of these molecules may prove to be appropriate anti-metastatic targets.

Cancer therapeutics has entered an era of molecular targeting. New agents are being developed to target specific molecular components on the cell surface or their downstream effectors that are important to tumor progression and survival. Signal transduction pathways such as the extracellular signal-regulated protein kinase/mitogen-activated protein kinase (ERK/MAPK) pathway have shown to be important for the pathogenesis of several cancers and inhibitors to specific molecules in this pathway have been developed and are in clinical trials (3, 4). Other agents have been developed for specific molecular defects. STI-571, an inhibitor of BCR-ABL tyrosine kinase, is used to treat chronic myeloid leukemia (5, 6). Monoclonal antibody therapy has also been employed with some success. Rituxan, an anti-CD-20 monoclonal antibody, has been approved for the treatment of B-cell lymphoma (7, 8). Herceptin, a monoclonal antibody to the HER2-neu receptor is effective in treating HER2-positive breast cancer (9,10). It is conceivable that cancer therapy will evolve into individualized therapy, treatment regimens will be designed based on the molecular characteristics of individual tumors.

Integrins are attractive as a therapeutic target because they are sentinel cell surface molecules for a plethora of cellular functions critical to cancer progression including cell survival and motility (11-14). This characteristic is particularly important in regard to cancer metastasis because integrins serve directly as a mediator for extracellular adhesion events necessary in metastasis while also integrating information from the extracellular environment into cellular signals that are required for cell motility and survival at distant sites in the body. The integrins $\alpha6\beta1$, $\alpha3\beta1$, and $\alpha6\beta4$ are associated with the progression of several epithelial tumors such as prostate, colon, breast, and pancreatic carcinomas (15-18). These laminin receptors are key to the understanding of the biology of cancer progression and may provide a foundation for therapeutic intervention to prevent metastasis.

Prostate cancer is an ideal malignancy to study genetic and protein changes that occur during progression to metastatic disease due to the fact that it is an indolent cancer and requires a long period of latency before metastatic conversion (19). Alterations that occur in integrin expression during prostate cancer progression has been extensively studied and seem to be early events (15, 20, 21). Complete loss of specific alpha and beta subunits are described and include α5, α4, αv, β1C, and β4 (15, 22, 23). Coupled with these findings, conservation of the integrins α6β1 and α3β1 have been documented (15, 21), making these laminin receptors critical molecular components and targets encompassing prostate cancer metastasis. The role of alpha-6 integrins has been solidified by the findings that α6β1 expression is maintained in prostate micrometastases (24). Taken together, these findings warrant further study of the biology of α6β1 during prostate cancer progression.

2. ISOLATION OF TUMOR CELL ADHESION PEPTIDES USING COMBINATORIAL PEPTIDE CHEMISTRY

The field of combinatorial peptide chemistry has enabled the creation of peptide ligand mimetics to multiple protein targets including kinases and cell surface receptors (reviewed in (25)). Combinatorial peptide chemistry allows the screening for peptide ligands among billions of random peptides created through a variety of approaches. The one-bead-one-compound combinatorial library method (26-29) and the phage-display peptide library approach (30-33) have been successfully used to identify peptide ligands for cell surface molecules. Isolation and characterization of these peptides not only creates potential inhibitors to their targets, it also fosters increased understanding of protein biology and function. This section will briefly compare the phage-display method to the OBOC approach and highlight the methodology behind the one-bead-one-compound combinatorial library for the development of tumor cell adhesion peptides.

2.1 Phage-Display Method

Phage-display is a biological library method that manipulates filamentous phage to display peptides on specific surface proteins such as the viral pIII coat protein located on one end of the phage (34). Random deoxyoligonucleotides dictating peptide size and orientation are inserted directly into the pIII gene creating a distinct peptide on the surface of individual phage (34). A few common methods are used to screen for peptides that bind to cell surface proteins such as panning for peptides with specificity to a cell surface protein by using purified cell surface receptors (35) or live cells (36, 37). Additionally, *in vivo* selection techniques have been developed by intravenous injection of phage-display libraries (38). Bound phages are collected and the amino acid sequence of the peptide displayed on each phagemid clone can be determined by DNA sequencing. Phage-display method has been applied successfully to identify peptide ligands against several integrins (39-41). Although this approach is limited to the use of L-amino acids, it is a powerful technique because up to 10^9 peptides can be screened per library while there is little restriction on the size of peptide displayed.

2.2 One-Bead-One-Compound Method

The one-bead-one-compound (OBOC) combinatorial method uses a solid phase technique and a "split-mix" synthesis approach to create a peptide library (26, 42 ,43). In essence, individual peptides are synthesized on polyethylene glycol-grafted polystyrene beads that yield approximately 10^{13} copies of the same peptide per bead (26, 27). Like the phage display method, OBOC libraries can identify cell surface ligands using purified receptors (27) or intact cells (44). One major advantage of the OBOC approach is that D-amino acids, unnatural amino acids or even nonamino acid moieties can be incorporated into OBOC libraries, whereas phages only display L-amino acid containing peptides. This is important for therapeutic purposes because peptides created for example, from D-amino acids are much more resistant to proteolysis *in vivo* (45, 46) and are therefore may have improved bioavailability and potency.

The OBOC approach has identified peptide ligand mimetics to different integrin heterodimers (47-49). We have used the OBOC peptide library method to identify peptide sequences that support tumor cell adhesion via the alpha-6 integrin (44, 50). The method of selection was based on functional cell adhesion of live tumor cells to peptide-containing beads. Briefly, DU-145H cells, a prostate tumor cell line that expresses high levels of $\alpha6$ (51), were applied to OBOC libraries and analyzed under a dissecting microscope. Beads with cells attached were retrieved, and those beads were rescreened with the same tumor cell line in the presence of a functional-blocking antibody to $\alpha6$, GoH3. The beads that no longer bound to tumor cells in this condition contained candidate $\alpha6$-specific adhesion peptides. Those beads were isolated, retested for adhesion without the antibody, and sequenced. Figure 1 displays the strategy for the selection of a cell adhesion peptide using the OBOC method. This method is particularly powerful because it does not require purification of the receptor and thus allows the appropriate post-translational modifications. In addition, by using live cells in this scheme, peptides can be identified that interact with conformationally sensitive surface molecules. In principle, this method allows the identification of specific cell adhesion peptides for any cell surface receptor for which a function-blocking reagent is available.

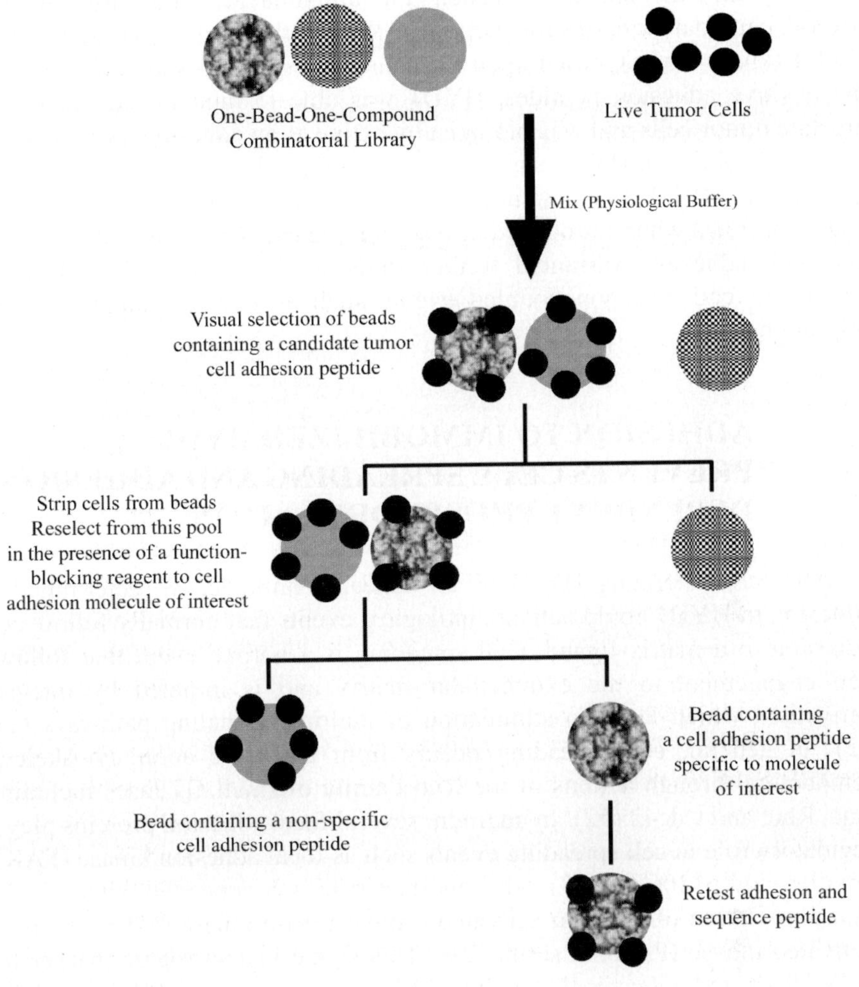

Figure 1. Isolation of tumor cell adhesion peptides using a one-bead-one-compound combinatorial library. The screen is based on functional cell adhesion. Tumor cells are incubated with a one-bead-one-compound combinatorial library in a column at 37°C for 90 minutes. The library is washed and examined with a dissecting microscope to visualize beads that directly bind to tumor cells. Positive beads are selected and stripped of cells with 0.1M HCl. These beads are screened again in the presence of a function-blocking reagent to the cell adhesion protein of interest. Consequently, the beads that do not bind to tumor cells may contain a peptide that interacts specifically with the cell adhesion protein of interest. These beads are retested to assure their ability to bind to tumor cells and sequenced to identify the peptide ligand. This selection scheme was used to isolate and characterize peptides that interact with α6 integrins (44, 50). Our scheme utilized the function-blocking antibody to α6, GoH3. This technique is powerful because it can identify candidate cell adhesion peptides to any adhesion protein with a function-blocking reagent available.

Using this method we screened a D-amino acid library that yielded several candidate α6-specific peptides. We synthesized a hybrid peptide, HYD1 (kikmviswkg), based upon the conserved sequences identified within the positive adhesion peptides. HYD1 was able to bind to the surface of prostate tumor cells and was biologically active as an adhesion mimetic (50). When immobilized, HYD1 supports integrin dependent tumor cell adhesion. In addition, HYD1 blocks tumor cell adhesion to immobilized extracellular matrix proteins when introduced as a soluble ligand. The ability of HYD1 to alter cell adhesion warranted further study to determine if HYD1 is an agonist to cell adhesion coupled events such as cell spreading and cell migration.

3. ADHESION TO IMMOBILIZED HYD1 PREVENTS CELL SPREADING AND ADHESION DEPENDENT PHOSPHORYLATION

After characterizing HYD1 as an adhesion mimetic, we determined if adhesion to HYD1 could activate biological events that normally follow cell adhesion to a matrix ligand. Cell spreading is a normal event that follows cell engagement to the extracellular matrix and is initiated by integrin activation, which leads to stimulation of multiple signaling pathways (14, 52). In general, cell spreading occurs from extensive actin cytoskeletal remodeling through actions of the Rho Family of small GTPases including Rac, Rho, and Cdc42 (52). In addition, several focal adhesion proteins play a regulatory role in cell spreading events such as focal adhesion kinase (FAK), paxillin, and p130CAS (53). An important adhesion dependent signal is the phosphorylation of mitogen activated protein kinase kinase (MEK) by p21-activated kinase (PAK) at serine 298. This signal is a surrogate marker for active PAK and indicates Rac activity (54).

To determine if HYD1 is a sufficient ligand to initiate cell spreading, we quantified the amount of cell spreading and average area occupied by the cells after adhesion to immobilized HYD1 or laminin-5 after 1 hour. As expected, adhesion to laminin-5 initiates cell spreading in nearly 100% of the cells within a microscopic field (Figure 2A). Interestingly, adhesion to HYD1 prevented cell spreading even in the presence of epithelial growth factor (EGF) (10ng/ml) (Figure 2B) suggesting that adhesion to immobilized HYD1 uncouples integrin-dependent adhesion from cell spreading.

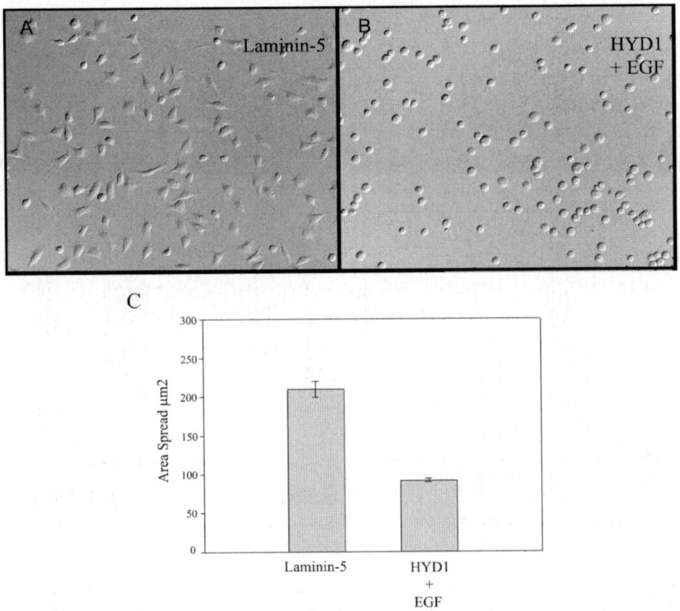

Figure 2. Adhesion to immobilized HYD1 prevents cell spreading. Spreading of PC3N cells (75), a variant of the prostate carcinoma cell line PC3 isolated from a bone metastasis, was determined using differential interference contrast optics on an inverted Olympus IMT2 microscope. A) PC3N cell spreading on a native ECM ligand, laminin 5, after 1 hour. B) PC3N cell spreading on HYD1 (150µg) + EGF 10ng/ml after 1 hour. C) Cell spreading was quantified with Compix Imaging software. Error bars are standard error from the mean area spread of 15 cells/experiment.

Since cell spreading events are tightly regulated by intracellular signals (52,53), we examined two integrin-proximal cellular signals that occurred during adhesion to HYD1. Adhesion to HYD1 induced phosphorylation of FAK on tyrosine 397 and MEK on serine 298 after thirty minutes of attachment (Figure 3A and B). The magnitude of the response was quite different when compared to cells attached to laminin-5 over the same time course (Figure 3A and B). Laminin-5 induced a robust activation of FAK at both 10 and 30 minutes post-adhesion while inducing significantly more phosphorylation of MEK at 10 minutes post-adhesion. Adhesion to HYDS (wiksmkivkg), a scrambled derivative of HYD1, was not able to induce a comparable response with either signal. Taken together these data suggest that adhesion to immobilized HYD1 uncouples cellular adhesion from cell spreading in part by suppressing normal adhesion dependent phosphorylation events.

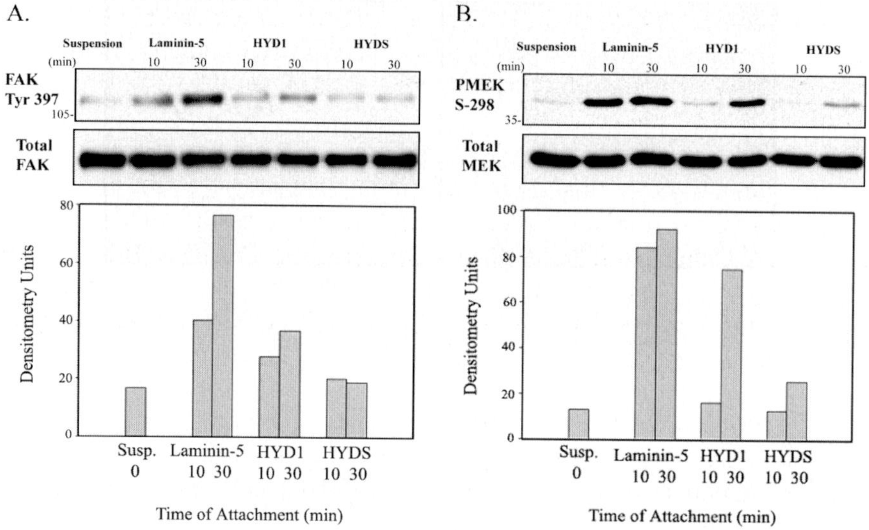

Figure 3. Suppression of adhesion dependent phosphorylation by immobilized HYD1. Phosphorylation of focal adhesion kinase (FAK) on tyrosine 397 (A) and the mitogen-activated protein kinase MEK1 on serine 298 (B) was analyzed by Western blot using phosphorylation specific antibodies. Densitometry analysis of percent phosphorylation is shown. PC3N cells were incubated in serum-free media overnight and attached in serum-free conditions to the indicated ligands for 10 and 30 minutes. Peptides were coated at a concentration of 150μg/plate. HYDS is a scrambled peptide derivative of HYD1.

4. CONCLUSION

There is a definite need for the development of novel agents that can block metastasis. Integrins specific for laminins are prime targets because they are involved directly in the mechanism of cell motility as well as providing an adhesion event crucial for cell survival and angiogenesis (11, 14). There are currently several integrin inhibitors under investigation for cancer therapy. Antagonists to αvβ3 and αvβ5 have been developed as antibody and peptide-based inhibitors to target angiogenesis and metastasis (55, 56). Vitaxin, a humanized αvβ3 antibody, is currently in Phase II trials (57-60). Cilengitide, a peptide inhibitor of αvβ3/αvβ5, is in Phase II trial for advanced solid tumors and has shown promise for use in combination therapy (61-64). In addition, other αvβ3 and α5β1-blocking peptides have been documented but have not yet entered clinical trials (65, 66). A humanized antibody has also been developed for α5β1 integrin, the fibronectin receptor, to target angiogenesis and is entering a Phase I trial (www.pdl.com). Although the current integrin-based therapeutics are promising, they are focused on αv and α5 integrin heterodimers. Antagonists to other integrins, specifically the laminin receptors, are likely to be equally beneficial.

We have used the one-bead-one-compound combinatorial method to isolate laminin receptor specific cell adhesion peptides. HYD1 (kikmviswkg), a candidate α6-integrin cell adhesion peptide, displays both agonist and antagonist effects on integrin function (50, 67). HYD1 is an adhesion agonist when immobilized yet uncouples the adhesion event from a cell spreading response. The most likely cause is due to the fact that the peptide did not initiate the identical signaling program as the native extracellular matrix. One explanation could be that the immobilized peptide lacks the proper avidity for integrin activation. Alternatively, HYD1 could initiate a signaling response that antagonizes particular integrin functions. This explanation is particularly intriguing because cell spreading was not induced on immobilized HYD1 even in the presence of the scatter factor EGF, suggesting that insufficient signaling may not be the primary mechanism for the lack of cell spreading following adhesion to HYD1. The ability of HYD1 to interrupt the normal response following cell adhesion may prove useful in developing agents to block cell invasion and metastasis or to control normal processes of tissue remodeling such as wound healing.

Combinatorial library methods, such as the one-bead-one-compound approach, have been successful in identifying and characterizing cell adhesion peptides with potential antagonistic effects on the targeted cell surface receptor. An argument against the use of peptide-based drugs is their poor bioavailability (56, 68, 69). However, modifications to increase bioavailability and potency have been applied to the cell adhesion peptides RGD and YIGSR with some success (70-72). In addition, using the peptide backbone as a template, chemical modifications can create pseudo-peptide analogs with increased stability and activity (73, 74). Therefore, the power of combinatorial library techniques such as the one-bead-one-compound approach should be harnessed to identify novel inhibitors of metastasis.

REFERENCES

1. Chambers, A.F., MacDonald, I.C., Schmidt, E.E., Morris, V.L., and Groom, A.C. (2000) Clinical targets for anti-metastasis therapy. Advances in Cancer Research, 79, 91-121.
2. Chambers, A.F., Groom, A.C., and MacDonald, I.C. (2002) Dissemination and growth of cancer cells in metastatic sites. Nat Rev Cancer, 2, 563-72.
3. Rinehart, J., Adjei, A.A., Lorusso, P.M., Waterhouse, D., Hecht, J.R., Natale, R.B., Hamid, O., Varterasian, M., Asbury, P., Kaldjian, E.P., Gulyas, S., Mitchell, D.Y., Herrera, R., Sebolt-Leopold, J.S., and Meyer, M.B. (2004) Multicenter phase II study of

the oral MEK inhibitor, CI-1040, in patients with advanced non-small-cell lung, breast, colon, and pancreatic cancer. J Clin Oncol, 22, 4456-62.
4. Allen, L.F., Sebolt-Leopold, J., and Meyer, M.B. (2003) CI-1040 (PD184352), a targeted signal transduction inhibitor of MEK (MAPKK). Semin Oncol, 30, 105-16.
5. Druker, B.J., Talpaz, M., Resta, D.J., Peng, B., Buchdunger, E., Ford, J.M., Lydon, N.B., Kantarjian, H., Capdeville, R., Ohno-Jones, S., and Sawyers, C.L. (2001) Efficacy and safety of a specific inhibitor of the BCR-ABL tyrosine kinase in chronic myeloid leukemia. N Engl J Med, 344, 1031-7.
6. Mauro, M.J. and Druker, B.J. (2001) STI571: targeting BCR-ABL as therapy for CML. Oncologist, 6, 233-8.
7. White, C.A., Larocca, A., and Grillo-Lopez, A.J. (1999) Anti-CD20 monoclonal antibodies as novel treatments for non-Hodgkin's lymphoma. Pharm. Sci. Technol. Today, 2, 95-101.
8. Grillo-Lopez, A.J., White, C.A., Varns, C., Shen, D., Wei, A., McClure, A., and Dallaire, B.K. (1999) Overview of the clinical development of rituximab: first monoclonal antibody approved for the treatment of lymphoma. Semin Oncol, 26, 66-73.
9. Dillman, R.O. (1999) Perceptions of Herceptin: a monoclonal antibody for the treatment of breast cancer. Cancer Biother Radiopharm, 14, 5-10.
10. Graziano, C. (1998) HER-2 breast assay, linked to Herceptin, wins FDA's okay. CAP Today, 12, 1, 14-6.
11. Jin, H. and Varner, J. (2004) Integrins: roles in cancer development and as treatment targets. Br J Cancer, 90, 561-5.
12. Hynes, R. (2002) Integrins: bidirectional, allosteric signaling machines. Cell, 110, 673-87.
13. Hood, J.D. and Cheresh, D.A. (2002) Role of integrins in cell invasion and migration. Nat Rev Cancer, 2, 91-100.
14. Hynes, R.O. (2002) Integrins: bidirectional, allosteric signaling machines. Cell, 110, 673-87.
15. Cress, A.E., Rabinovitz, I., Zhu, W., and Nagle, R.B. (1995) The alpha 6 beta 1 and alpha 6 beta 4 integrins in human prostate cancer progression. Cancer Metastasis Rev, 14, 219-28.
16. Friedrichs, K., Ruiz, P., Franke, F., Gille, I., Terpe, H.J., and Imhof, B.A. (1995) High expression level of alpha 6 integrin in human breast carcinoma is correlated with reduced survival. Cancer Res, 55, 901-6.
17. Rabinovitz, I. and Mercurio, A.M. (1996) The integrin alpha 6 beta 4 and the biology of carcinoma. Biochem Cell Biol, 74, 811-21.
18. Rosendahl, A., Neumann, K., Chaloupka, B., Rothmund, M., and Weinel, R.J. (1993) Expression and distribution of VLA receptors in the pancreas: an immunohistochemical study. Pancreas, 8, 711-8.
19. Johansson, J.E., Andren, O., Andersson, S.O., Dickman, P.W., Holmberg, L., Magnuson, A., and Adami, H.O. (2004) Natural history of early, localized prostate cancer. Jama, 291, 2713-9.
20. Banyard, J. and Zetter, B.R. (1998) The role of cell motility in prostate cancer. Cancer Metastasis Rev, 17, 449-58.
21. Nagle, R.B., Hao, J., Knox, J.D., Dalkin, B.L., Clark, V., and Cress, A.E. (1995) Expression of hemidesmosomal and extracellular matrix proteins by normal and malignant human prostate tissue. Am J Pathol, 146, 1498-507.

22. Fornaro, M., Tallini, G., Bofetiado, C.J., Bosari, S., and Languino, L.R. (1996) Down-regulation of beta 1C integrin, an inhibitor of cell proliferation, in prostate carcinoma. Am J Pathol, 149, 765-73.
23. Perlino, E., Lovecchio, M., Vacca, R.A., Fornaro, M., Moro, L., Ditonno, P., Battaglia, M., Selvaggi, F.P., Mastropasqua, M.G., Bufo, P., and Languino, L.R. (2000) Regulation of mRNA and protein levels of beta1 integrin variants in human prostate carcinoma. Am J Pathol, 157, 1727-34.
24. Putz, E., Witter, K., Offner, S., Stosiek, P., Zippelius, A., Johnson, J., Zahn, R., Riethmuller, G., and Pantel, K. (1999) Phenotypic characteristics of cell lines derived from disseminated cancer cells in bone marrow of patients with solid epithelial tumors: establishment of working models for human micrometastases. Cancer Res, 59, 241-8.
25. Liu, R., Enstrom, A.M., and Lam, K.S. (2003) Combinatorial peptide library methods for immunobiology research. Exp Hematol, 31, 11-30.
26. Lam, K.S., Salmon, S.E., Hersh, E.M., Hruby, V.J., Kazmierski, W.M., and Knapp, R.J. (1991) A new type of synthetic peptide library for identifying ligand-binding activity. Nature, 354, 82-4.
27. Lam, K.S., Lebl, M., and Krchnak, V. (1997) The "One-Bead-One-Compound" Combinatorial Library Method. Chem Rev, 97, 411-448.
28. Lam, K.S., Liu, R., Miyamoto, S., Lehman, A.L., and Tuscano, J.M. (2003) Applications of one-bead one-compound combinatorial libraries and chemical microarrays in signal transduction research. Acc Chem Res, 36, 370-7.
29. Wang, X., Peng, L., Liu, R., Xu, B., and Lam, K.S. (2005) Applications of topologically segregated bilayer beads in 'one-bead one-compound' combinatorial libraries. J Pept Res, 65, 130-8.
30. Cwirla, S.E., Peters, E.A., Barrett, R.W., and Dower, W.J. (1990) Peptides on phage: a vast library of peptides for identifying ligands. Proc Natl Acad Sci U S A, 87, 6378-82.
31. Devlin, J.J., Panganiban, L.C., and Devlin, P.E. (1990) Random peptide libraries: a source of specific protein binding molecules. Science, 249, 404-6.
32. Rodi, D.J., Makowski, L., and Kay, B.K. (2002) One from column A and two from column B: the benefits of phage display in molecular-recognition studies. Curr Opin Chem Biol, 6, 92-6.
33. Trepel, M., Arap, W., and Pasqualini, R. (2002) In vivo phage display and vascular heterogeneity: implications for targeted medicine. Curr Opin Chem Biol, 6, 399-404.
34. Parmley, S.F. and Smith, G.P. (1988) Antibody-selectable filamentous fd phage vectors: affinity purification of target genes. Gene, 73, 305-18.
35. Fukuda, M.N., Ohyama, C., Lowitz, K., Matsuo, O., Pasqualini, R., Ruoslahti, E., and Fukuda, M. (2000) A peptide mimic of E-selectin ligand inhibits sialyl Lewis X-dependent lung colonization of tumor cells. Cancer Res, 60, 450-6.
36. Romanov, V.I., Durand, D.B., and Petrenko, V.A. (2001) Phage display selection of peptides that affect prostate carcinoma cells attachment and invasion. Prostate, 47, 239-51.
37. Zhang, J., Spring, H., and Schwab, M. (2001) Neuroblastoma tumor cell-binding peptides identified through random peptide phage display. Cancer Lett, 171, 153-64.
38. Kolonin, M., Pasqualini, R., and Arap, W. (2001) Molecular addresses in blood vessels as targets for therapy. Curr Opin Chem Biol, 5, 308-13.
39. Murayama, O., Nishida, H., and Sekiguchi, K. (1996) Novel peptide ligands for integrin alpha 6 beta 1 selected from a phage display library. J Biochem (Tokyo), 120, 445-51.

40. Koivunen, E., Wang, B., and Ruoslahti, E. (1995) Phage libraries displaying cyclic peptides with different ring sizes: ligand specificities of the RGD-directed integrins. Biotechnology (N Y), 13, 265-70.
41. Assa-Munt, N., Jia, X., Laakkonen, P., and Ruoslahti, E. (2001) Solution structures and integrin binding activities of an RGD peptide with two isomers. Biochemistry, 40, 2373-8.
42. Houghten, R.A., Pinilla, C., Blondelle, S.E., Appel, J.R., Dooley, C.T., and Cuervo, J.H. (1991) Generation and use of synthetic peptide combinatorial libraries for basic research and drug discovery. Nature, 354, 84-6.
43. Furka, A., Sebestyen, F., Asgedom, M., and Dibo, G. (1991) General method for rapid synthesis of multicomponent peptide mixtures. Int J Pept Protein Res, 37, 487-93.
44. Pennington, M.E., Lam, K.S., and Cress, A.E. (1996) The use of a combinatorial library method to isolate human tumor cell adhesion peptides. Mol Divers, 2, 19-28.
45. Hamamoto, K., Kida, Y., Zhang, Y., Shimizu, T., and Kuwano, K. (2002) Antimicrobial activity and stability to proteolysis of small linear cationic peptides with D-amino acid substitutions. Microbiol Immunol, 46, 741-9.
46. Van Regenmortel, M.H. and Muller, S. (1998) D-peptides as immunogens and diagnostic reagents. Curr Opin Biotechnol, 9, 377-82.
47. Aina, O.H., Marik, J., Liu, R., Lau, D.H., and Lam, K.S. (2005) Identification of novel targeting peptides for human ovarian cancer cells using "one-bead one-compound" combinatorial libraries. Mol Cancer Ther, 4, 806-13.
48. Lau, D.H., Guo, L.L, Liu, R.W., Song, A.M., Shao, C.K., and Lam, K.S. (2002) Identifying peptide ligands for cell surface receptors using cell-growth-on-bead-assay and one-bead-one-compound combinatorial library. Biotechnology Letters, 24, 497-500.
49. Park S.I., R.M., Vikstrom, B., Amro, N., Song, L., Xu, B., and Lam K.S. (2002) The use of one-bead one-compound combinatorial library method to identify peptide ligands for Alpha4Beta1 integrin receptor in non-Hodgkin's lymphoma. Letters in Peptide Science, 8, 171-178.
50. DeRoock, I.B., Pennington, M.E., Sroka, T.C., Lam, K.S., Bowden, G.T., Bair, E.L., and Cress, A.E. (2001) Synthetic peptides inhibit adhesion of human tumor cells to extracellular matrix proteins. Cancer Res, 61, 3308-13.
51. Rabinovitz, I., Nagle, R.B., and Cress, A.E. (1995) Integrin alpha 6 expression in human prostate carcinoma cells is associated with a migratory and invasive phenotype in vitro and in vivo. Clin Exp Metastasis, 13, 481-91.
52. Arthur, W.T., Noren, N.K., and Burridge, K. (2002) Regulation of Rho family GTPases by cell-cell and cell-matrix adhesion. Biol Res, 35, 239-46.
53. Panetti, T.S. (2002) Tyrosine phosphorylation of paxillin, FAK, and p130CAS: effects on cell spreading and migration. Front Biosci, 7, d143-50.
54. Slack-Davis, J.K., Eblen, S.T., Zecevic, M., Boerner, S.A., Tarcsafalvi, A., Diaz, H.B., Marshall, M.S., Weber, M.J., Parsons, J.T., and Catling, A.D. (2003) PAK1 phosphorylation of MEK1 regulates fibronectin-stimulated MAPK activation. J Cell Biol, 162, 281-91.
55. Kerr, J.S., Slee, A.M., and Mousa, S.A. (2002) The alpha v integrin antagonists as novel anticancer agents: an update. Expert Opin Investig Drugs, 11, 1765-74.
56. Tucker, G.C. (2003) Alpha v integrin inhibitors and cancer therapy. Curr Opin Investig Drugs, 4, 722-31.
57. Gutheil, J.C., Campbell, T.N., Pierce, P.R., Watkins, J.D., Huse, W.D., Bodkin, D.J., and Cheresh, D.A. (2000) Targeted antiangiogenic therapy for cancer using Vitaxin: a

humanized monoclonal antibody to the integrin alphavbeta3. Clin Cancer Res, 6, 3056-61.

58. Mikecz, K. (2000) Vitaxin applied molecular evolution. Curr Opin Investig Drugs, 1, 199-203.
59. Patel, S.R., Jenkins, J., Papadopolous, N., Burgess, M.A., Plager, C., Gutterman, J., and Benjamin, R.S. (2001) Pilot study of vitaxin--an angiogenesis inhibitor-in patients with advanced leiomyosarcomas. Cancer, 92, 1347-8.
60. Posey, J.A., Khazaeli, M.B., DelGrosso, A., Saleh, M.N., Lin, C.Y., Huse, W., and LoBuglio, A.F. (2001) A pilot trial of Vitaxin, a humanized anti-vitronectin receptor (anti alpha v beta 3) antibody in patients with metastatic cancer. Cancer Biother Radiopharm, 16, 125-32.
61. Smith, J.W. (2003) Cilengitide Merck. Curr Opin Investig Drugs, 4, 741-5.
62. Eskens, F.A., Dumez, H., Hoekstra, R., Perschl, A., Brindley, C., Bottcher, S., Wynendaele, W., Drevs, J., Verweij, J., and van Oosterom, A.T. (2003) Phase I and pharmacokinetic study of continuous twice weekly intravenous administration of Cilengitide (EMD 121974), a novel inhibitor of the integrins alphavbeta3 and alphavbeta5 in patients with advanced solid tumours. Eur J Cancer, 39, 917-26.
63. Burke, P.A., DeNardo, S.J., Miers, L.A., Lamborn, K.R., Matzku, S., and DeNardo, G.L. (2002) Cilengitide targeting of alpha(v)beta(3) integrin receptor synergizes with radioimmunotherapy to increase efficacy and apoptosis in breast cancer xenografts. Cancer Res, 62, 4263-72.
64. Raguse, J.D., Gath, H.J., Bier, J., Riess, H., and Oettle, H. (2004) Cilengitide (EMD 121974) arrests the growth of a heavily pretreated highly vascularised head and neck tumour. Oral Oncol, 40, 228-30.
65. Reinmuth, N., Liu, W., Ahmad, S.A., Fan, F., Stoeltzing, O., Parikh, A.A., Bucana, C.D., Gallick, G.E., Nickols, M.A., Westlin, W.F., and Ellis, L.M. (2003) Alphavbeta3 integrin antagonist S247 decreases colon cancer metastasis and angiogenesis and improves survival in mice. Cancer Res, 63, 2079-87.
66. Stoeltzing, O., Liu, W., Reinmuth, N., Fan, F., Parry, G.C., Parikh, A.A., McCarty, M.F., Bucana, C.D., Mazar, A.P., and Ellis, L.M. (2003) Inhibition of integrin alpha5beta1 function with a small peptide (ATN-161) plus continuous 5-FU infusion reduces colorectal liver metastases and improves survival in mice. Int J Cancer, 104, 496-503.
67. Sroka, Pennington, M.E., and Cress, A.E. (2005) Synthetic D-Amino Acid Peptide Inhibits Tumor Cell Motility on Laminin-5. Carcinogenesis, In Press.
68. Mahato, R.I., Narang, A.S., Thoma, L., and Miller, D.D. (2003) Emerging trends in oral delivery of peptide and protein drugs. Crit Rev Ther Drug Carrier Syst, 20, 153-214.
69. Hamman, J.H., Enslin, G.M., and Kotze, A.F. (2005) Oral delivery of Peptide drugs : barriers and developments. BioDrugs, 19, 165-77.
70. Kumagai, H., Tajima, M., Ueno, Y., Giga-Hama, Y., and Ohba, M. (1991) Effect of cyclic RGD peptide on cell adhesion and tumor metastasis. Biochem Biophys Res Commun, 177, 74-82.
71. Kaneda, Y., Yamamoto, Y., Okada, N., Tsutsuml, Y., Nakagawa, S., Kakiuch, M., Maeda, M., Kawasaki, K., and Mayumi, T. (1997) Antimetastatic effect of synthetic Glu-Ile-Leu-Asp-Val peptide derivatives containing D-amino acids. Anticancer Drugs, 8, 702-7.
72. Yamamoto, Y., Tsutsumi, Y., and Mayumi, T. (2002) Molecular design of bioconjugated cell adhesion peptide with a water-soluble polymeric modifier for enhancement of antimetastatic effect. Curr Drug Targets, 3, 123-30.

73. Fujii, H., Nishikawa, N., Komazawa, H., Suzuki, M., Kojima, M., Itoh, I., Obata, A., Ayukawa, K., Azuma, I., and Saiki, I. (1998) A new pseudo-peptide of Arg-Gly-Asp (RGD) with inhibitory effect on tumor metastasis and enzymatic degradation of extracellular matrix. Clin Exp Metastasis, 16, 94-104.
74. Dechantsreiter, M.A., Planker, E., Matha, B., Lohof, E., Holzemann, G., Jonczyk, A., Goodman, S.L., and Kessler, H. (1999) N-Methylated cyclic RGD peptides as highly active and selective alpha(V)beta(3) integrin antagonists. J Med Chem, 42, 3033-40.
75. Tran, N.L., Nagle, R.B., Cress, A.E., and Heimark, R.L. (1999) N-Cadherin expression in human prostate carcinoma cell lines. An epithelial-mesenchymal transformation mediating adhesion with Stromal cells. Am J Pathol, 155, 787-98.

Index